THE FACTS ABOUT PMS

DID YOU KNOW?

- The symptoms of PMS may change or grow more severe during different phases of your life.

- Every body system—from your nerves to your blood—can be affected by PMS.

- Vitamin therapy can lessen symptoms.

- Your self-image can influence whether or not you experience distress from PMS.

- PMS symptoms can mimic serious mental illness.

Knowing what is happening to your body is vitally important for every woman. You no longer have to be at the mercy of your hormones. This helpful, caring guide helps you control PMS with a long-range life-style program and gives you sound information about the most effective treatment for its physical and emotional effects.

RELIEF FROM PMS

THE DELL MEDICAL LIBRARY

THE DELL MEDICAL LIBRARY

Relief from
PMS

Pamela Patrick Novotny

*Foreword by Phillip S. Alberts, M.D.,
F.A.C.O.G.*

A LYNN SONBERG BOOK

Published by
Dell Publishing
a division of
Bantam Doubleday Dell Publishing Group, Inc.
666 Fifth Avenue
New York, New York 10103

Research about premenstrual syndrome is ongoing and subject
to interpretation. Although every effort has been made to
include the most up-to-date and accurate information in this
book, there can be no guarantee that what we know about this
complex subject won't change with time. The reader should
bear in mind that this book should not be used for self-
diagnosis or self-treatment and should consult appropriate
medical professionals regarding all health issues.

ISBN: 0-440-21086-0

Published by arrangement with Lynn Sonberg Book Services,
166 East 56 Street, 3-C, New York, NY 10022.

Printed in the United States of America

Published simultaneously in Canada

September 1992

10 9 8 7 6 5 4 3 2 1

OPM

ACKNOWLEDGMENTS

Sincere thanks to each of the following for their time, expertise, information, and assistance:

Phillip S. Alberts, M.D., F.A.C.O.G.
PMS Treatment Center
Portland, Oregon

American Academy of Family Physicians
Kansas City, Missouri

American College of Obstetricians and Gynecologists
Washington, D.C.

Michael S. Alberts, Ph.D., Medical Psychology
Oregon Health Sciences University and
  PMS Treatment Center
Portland, Oregon

Donald G. DeLong, M.D.
Alternative Medicine Foundation
Marina Del Rey, California

National Women's Health Network
Washington, D.C.

CONTENTS

FOREWORD

Every month millions of women feel the effects of premenstrual syndrome, PMS. For some, it means a few moody days. But for others, it's much more drastic, producing depression, weight gain, headaches, flare-ups of chronic conditions like asthma or herpes, and more.

If you are one of those women who spend several days each month wondering if you are going crazy, or if you dread those PMS days you know you'll spend feeling out of control, *Relief from PMS* offers hope.

While there are no miracle cures for PMS (and no one has even pinpointed a single cause for it), there are many approaches you can take to reduce or erase its symptoms. But before you embark on treatment, it's important that you understand the hormonal cycles that underlie PMS. That's where *Relief from PMS* comes in. Here you'll find a comprehensive description of all you need to know to understand your body and the systems that have a part in producing PMS symptoms.

In my own practice I see the patient, and often her family, too, as the key to correctly evaluating and diagnosing PMS. I've also found a multidisciplinary treatment program that includes counseling and education to be the most effective. Both these approaches are part of the basic premise from which *Relief from PMS* is written. Life-style changes that work, information about diet and exercise, hormone treatments, and even alternative approaches are all covered here. The book also offers help in finding the right physician or clinic for you and what should ideally happen in a qualified treatment program.

But perhaps most important, *Relief from PMS* does not address the woman who reads this book as deficient or diseased because of her very real monthly symptoms. Instead, it takes the view that if a woman understands how her body works and what she requires as a female, she will be able to take action to feel better.

Relief from PMS offers scores of actions. For the woman with PMS, it is a starting point on the road to relief.

PHILLIP S. ALBERTS, M.D., F.A.C.O.G.
Medical Director
PMS Treatment Center
Portland, Oregon

INTRODUCTION

If you think you have PMS—premenstrual syndrome—and you think there's nothing you can do about it, it's time to take another look.

True, there's no "magic formula" that will erase all your symptoms overnight, but as research progresses, more and more help is available.

In the first chapter of *Relief from PMS,* you'll see why PMS is such a difficult collection of symptoms to deal with. You'll get an overview of current theory about the causes of PMS and a look at how PMS symptoms differ for women depending on their age.

Once you have a clear understanding of PMS symptoms and where they may come from, Chapter 3 will help you begin charting your own symptoms so that when you see a physician you'll have the kind of information that will help him or her arrive at a diagnosis and a treatment plan. You'll also find descriptions of other conditions commonly mistaken for PMS.

For many women, the approach that works the best is the simplest: making life-style changes. Chapter 4 explains just how to do that, whether it's diet that needs correcting or a new exercise program you can start. Food supplements like vitamins, minerals, and herbs are discussed in Chapter 6, along with some alternative approaches like biofeedback.

If you and your physician see the medical route as most appropriate for you, Chapter 5 gives you the rundown on what works and for whom. From progesterone therapy to hysterectomies, all the major medical/surgical approaches are included.

Finally, even though PMS is most definitely not all in your head, there are ways of looking at it that you may find helpful as you journey toward understanding and control of its symptoms. Chapter 7 shows how in other cultures and other times women made allowances for their biology in ways we do not and how you may apply what they knew to your life.

Relief from PMS offers all the information and guidance you need to help you develop an individualized approach to your PMS symptoms. Read it, and feel saner and more able to handle the difficult days before your period.

ONE

WHAT IS PREMENSTRUAL SYNDROME?

- It had been a normal nine-to-five workday for Jill; no overtime this week. At home that evening she and Gary prepared dinner together; then she helped their daughter, Marcy, study her spelling words. While Gary read to Marcy and tucked her into bed, Jill balanced the checkbook. She turned in early, feeling pleasantly smug about the balanced account, cozy and content with her life. Why then, when Jill awoke the next morning, did she feel instantly depressed, too heavy to lift herself from the bed, annoyed with the everyday morning sounds of Gary chiding Marcy to get up? What had happened overnight to change her mood so drastically?

- Katie's menstrual period had started right after her twelfth birthday, and her mom had explained that it wasn't unusual for its date of arrival each month to be unpredictable at first. When Katie started complaining of feeling full and bloated just before her period and grouchy with her friends, her mother explained that was normal too. But when Katie asked what she could do about it, her mom only shrugged and shook her head.

• Usually Maryann felt good about how she cared for her two toddlers; she saw herself as caring, creative, patient. Other times she felt controlled by a raging anger that appeared out of nowhere. Then she felt she was watching herself create horrible scenes involving her husband and children that she was unable to stop. Maryann worried she'd hurt one of her children, and she was beginning to wonder if she had a personality disorder.

Different as they may seem, each of these women has premenstrual syndrome (PMS), a collection of symptoms shared by an estimated forty-five million American women.

WHAT IS PMS?

Until the early 1980s PMS wasn't recognized as a problem that existed apart from the imaginations of women, although it was first described in medical literature as early as the 1930s. Today, while PMS is seen as a legitimate condition, what health care providers don't know about it far outweighs what they do know. And they don't know the most basic of information, for no single cause has been identified so far. Consequently there is no single treatment that works for everyone.

That's the bad news. The good news is that a wide variety of treatments do work on various PMS symptoms for many women. And research is continuing to find out more.

The best way to understand PMS and how it affects you is to talk about symptoms. PMS is a biobehavioral problem, meaning that it has both psychological and physical components. So far there are about 150 symptoms, or components, identified with PMS. That's why it's called a syndrome, a collection of symptoms. These symptoms affect every system in the body, and it is as common for one woman to have one or two symptoms as it is to have ten or twelve.

Some of the physical symptoms of PMS are:

—headaches, migraines

—joint and muscle aches and swelling

—backaches

—food cravings, increased appetite, thirst, sugar cravings

—decreased alcohol tolerance

—clumsiness

—changes in sex drive

—constipation, diarrhea

—sweating, shakiness, dizziness, fainting

—hoarseness, sore throat

—cystitis, urethritis, less frequent urination

—abdominal bloating, weight gain

—acne, boils, hives, allergies

—breast tenderness and swelling

Some women also report that PMS makes worse certain chronic disorders, such as asthma, sinusitis, vaginal yeast infections, seizures, herpes, and allergies.

You may notice that cramping and abdominal pain are not on this list. Some people associate these with PMS, but in fact, they usually occur *during* the menstrual period rather than before it. There is a separate medical term for painful periods, dysmenorrhea, and it will not be covered here.

Some of the psychological symptoms of PMS are:

—loss of emotional control

—anxiety

—forgetfulness

—decreased concentration

—confusion

—withdrawal

—depression

—nightmares

—mood swings

—hostility, irritability

—loss of self-confidence

Estimates of how many women experience some of these symptoms vary widely. Some sources say *every* woman experiences at least one or two of these at some time. The American College of Obstetricians and Gynecologists has reported that about 20 to 40 percent of all women have some PMS symptoms, with about 5 to 7 percent of them having symptoms severe enough to affect their life-styles. At the other end of the spectrum one study showed that about 5 percent of women feel absolutely no psychological, emotional, or physical changes in themselves in the two weeks prior to their periods.

WHO HAS IT?

There is an inherent difficulty in talking about who has PMS and who doesn't because the condition has no standard definition. One woman may call a single day of irritability PMS; another may have five or six pounds of weight gain before her period and not consider herself a sufferer. Yet another may notice a surge of creativity in the last two weeks of her cycle; is that positive PMS?

While individual descriptions and perceptions of what constitutes PMS vary, most health care providers agree on two conditions that must exist before a woman is diagnosed with it:

—She must experience a cluster of *recurring* symptoms. While the same symptoms don't have to occur every month for them to constitute PMS, there must be a recurring pattern. Similar symptoms occurring every third month are typical for some women, for example.

—The symptoms must occur *at the right time*: during the week or two before her menstrual period, followed by a symptom-free phase each cycle. Typically, PMS symptoms fall into one of four time frames:

• They occur around ovulation for a day or two, then disappear until a couple of days before the period, lasting until about twenty-four hours after the period begins.

- They begin at ovulation and continue fairly consistently until twenty-four hours after menstrual bleeding has begun.

- They occur two to ten days before the beginning of menstrual bleeding and last about twenty-four hours into the period.

- They begin at ovulation and last all the way until the end of the menstrual period, a total of about three weeks.

Even though these patterns are typical for many women, yours may be different and still constitute PMS.

While PMS symptoms are most common in women between the ages of twenty-five and forty-five, they have been reported in some preteen girls who have such PMS-like symptoms as cyclical mood swings *before* menarche (their first-ever menstrual period) as well as in women who have had partial hysterectomies or who have entered menopause.

As with many aspects of PMS, no one knows for sure why some individuals seem more vulnerable to it than others, but some researchers theorize that you may be at increased risk for PMS if you:

—are over thirty. Many women report that symptoms worsen with age.

—use birth control pills or have just discontinued their use. Women at some PMS clinics report more serious symptoms while they are on or just coming off oral contraceptives.

—have just had a baby. Many women report first having
PMS, or having intensified symptoms of their old PMS,
when their period returns after the birth of a child.

—have had more than one pregnancy. More than half the
women seeking help for PMS at several clinics have
had two or more pregnancies (including abortions and
miscarriages).

—have had postpartum depression lasting more than ten
days.

—have a mother or sister with PMS. While no formal
research confirms this, many women seeking help for
PMS report that their mothers or sisters apparently
had/have it too.

—have just had a tubal ligation or a partial hysterectomy
(also known as a subtotal hysterectomy). Hormonal
fluctuations at these times are enough to trigger PMS
in some women.

—have recently been divorced or experienced the death
of someone close to you. Times of extreme
psychological stress can cause the same hormonal
fluctuations as certain physical stresses.

Some researchers believe more women today experience
PMS because they have more menstrual periods during
their lifetimes than did women in previous centuries and
consequently more opportunity to feel PMS symptoms.
They see two reasons for this:

—Women menstruate for more years overall most likely
because of better nutrition and living conditions. Prior
to this century the average age for a girl's first period

was fourteen, and her last occurred around age forty. Now in the United States the average age for menarche is around eleven or twelve, and menopause occurs on average during a woman's early fifties.

—Women spend less time pregnant and/or breast-feeding than women did in the past and thus have many more years of uninterrupted menstruation. For example, if you followed the typical pattern of a nineteenth-century woman, giving birth to a child every two years and breast-feeding for most of the months between pregnancies, you might have only one or two menstrual periods a year. It's hard to establish a feel for PMS symptoms when you menstruate only once a year. But your experience with menstruation, and PMS, is very different if you have uninterrupted periods for fifteen years until you are in your thirties, have one or two children, and then menstruate uninterruptedly again until menopause.

THE PSYCHOLOGICAL IMPACT OF PMS

Many women who seek help at PMS clinics report that the physical symptoms they feel are secondary to the psychological distress that PMS can bring. Feelings of being out of control and unable to hold back tears or angry outbursts, of living inside a cloud of depression, confusion, and anxiety all are blows to self-esteem.

Considering that so many women are working hard to strike a balance between job and family responsibilities—a stressful situation in itself—it is not surprising that PMS symptoms, in addition to all the "normal" stresses, can be especially devastating. Michelle Harrison, M.D., who wrote

Self-Help for Premenstrual Syndrome, notes, "Women who say they feel 'crazy' premenstrually often have good reason to feel that way." She suggests that most women could begin mitigating the psychological stresses in their lives, and eventually the PMS stress, by giving themselves credit for all they do. Whether it's meeting a deadline at work or shepherding two toddlers as you run errands, it's helpful to pat yourself on the back for accomplishing tasks that some would find overwhelming at any time of the month.

Changing expectations of ourselves to accommodate monthly cycles is one way of coping with PMS. But understanding how your menstrual cycle works is the first step. The next chapter leads you through the steps of the cycle and the hormones, glands, and organs that make it work.

WHERE PMS BEGINS

As the last chapter explained, premenstrual syndrome is a collection of symptoms that affect some women during the two weeks preceding their menstrual periods. To understand the symptoms and what to do about them, it is first important to understand menstruation.

Several organs and glands work together each month to produce a period. In the section below, the functions of these glands and organs will be explained by tracing:

—the messages carried to them by chemical substances called hormones

—the journey of the egg the hormones produce

—the path of the menstrual blood and tissue as they flow to the outside of the body

The section in this chapter entitled "The Menstrual Cycle" will explain in further detail how hormones affect the cycle as well as physical and emotional well-being.

ORGANS AND GLANDS

Each menstrual cycle begins with the endocrine glands in your brain, the hypothalamus and the pituitary.

Hypothalamus. Beneath the cerebral cortex of the brain lies the hypothalamus. Exactly how it carries out its functions (among others, it produces beta-endorphins—the "feel-good" hormones or opiates—and controls appetite, body temperature, emotional integration, and the menstrual cycle) is not completely understood. We know that the hypothalamus receives from the brain signals that trigger its secretion of gonadotropin-releasing hormone (GnRH) into tiny blood vessels that lead to the pituitary.

Pituitary. If you could follow a line from the bridge of your nose directly back to the base of your brain, you would come across the pituitary. It is within this tiny gland, which is less than one-half inch in diameter, that follicle-stimulating hormone (FSH) and luteinizing hormone (LH) are synthesized and stored. Messages from the hypothalamus in the form of GnRH stimulate the release of these hormones at different times during the menstrual cycle. FSH and LH in turn send messages to the ovaries that trigger the maturation of oocytes (immature eggs), the production of estrogen, and the release of eggs from the ovaries.

Ovaries. The two ovaries, which are attached by thin stalks to the uterus on either side near its top, are about walnut size. The ovaries produce estrogen and progesterone and release one mature egg, or ovum, each menstrual cycle.

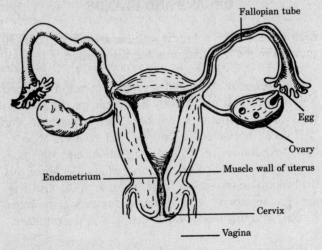

Female reproductive organs

Fallopian Tubes. Also attached near the top of the uterus are these two sturdy tubes, one on each side. Each tube, or oviduct, is about four inches long, the free end opening out like a trumpet with tiny waving tendrils called fimbriae hovering near the ovaries. When a mature egg bursts from the ovary, it is caught by the fimbriae and moved down the inside of the tube toward the uterus by the tube's lubricating mucous membrane and by beating, hair-like cilia.

Uterus. After the egg has traveled down the Fallopian tube, it comes to the uterus, a pear-shaped muscular organ. The uterus is lined with another kind of mucous membrane, called the endometrium, which changes with the type of hormone being secreted by the ovaries, the hypothalamus, and the pituitary. Hormones stimulate the endometrium to create tissue and to increase the blood supply to this new tissue so that it can nurture a fertilized egg. If the egg that comes into the uterus is not fertilized and does not implant in the endometrium, the egg and the extra tissue and blood are shed during a menstrual period.

Cervix. At the narrow base of the uterus, the cervix is a fibrous ring of tissue with a tiny opening, called the os, which allows menstrual fluid to flow out to the vagina. The cervix also holds many mucous glands that secrete different kinds of mucus depending on the kind of hormone being produced in the woman's body.

Vagina. This is the passage between the uterus and the protective folds of the vulva on the outside of the body. It is a strong, mucous-membrane-lined organ about three to five inches long through which menstrual blood and discarded tissue flow to the outside of the body.

THE MENSTRUAL CYCLE

The length of the menstrual cycle is different for each woman, but twenty-eight days is the average. It's important to understand that the twenty-eight-day cycle is the idealized version and that however long *your* cycle is, it is the correct length for you.

There are four distinct hormonal phases in the menstrual cycle:

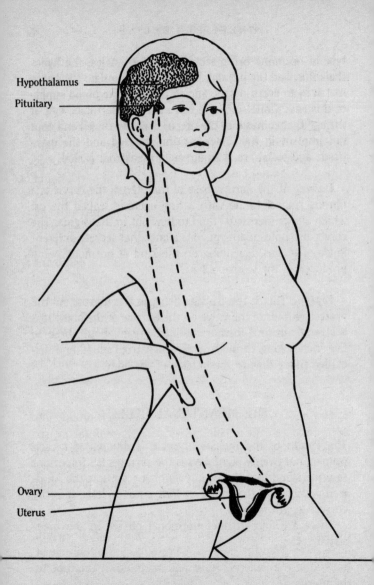

Hypothalamus

Pituitary

Ovary

Uterus

Hormones and the menstural cycle

1. *Follicular phase.* This begins with the first day of menstrual bleeding, called Day 1 of your cycle. At about Day 5 your brain reports low estrogen levels to the hypothalamus, which sends GnRH to the pituitary.

The pituitary responds by sending out FSH (follicle-stimulating hormone), which causes oocytes to begin developing in each ovary and stimulates the ovaries to produce estrogen. A single follicle, usually the first to develop and the largest, soon becomes dominant.

In response to the increased estrogen being produced by the ovaries and the dominant follicle, the pituitary slows its output of FSH. Now the smaller, less developed follicles can't get enough FSH, so they die off, leaving the dominant follicle to absorb all the FSH and produce estrogen.

Just in case the egg in the follicle is soon fertilized, increased amounts of estrogen cause the endometrium to form a new blanket of cells supplied with oxygen and nutrients by tiny arteries. The endometrium grows so much that by mid-cycle, or around Day 14, it is three times as thick as it was on Day 1 and has a greatly increased blood supply.

2. *Ovulation.* By about Day 13 or 14 estrogen production from the dominant follicle has reached its peak (about six times what it was on Day 1) and remains there for about forty-eight hours. In response, the hypothalamus releases GnRH to the pituitary, which releases a surge of LH (luteinizing hormone).

After about twenty-four hours of LH surge, the wall of the follicle disintegrates, and the dominant egg, or ovum, floats away from the ovary to be caught by the fimbriae at the end of the Fallopian tube and swept down the tube to the uterus.

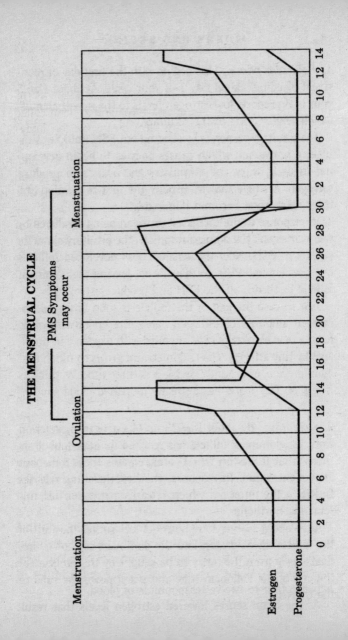

THE MENSTRUAL CYCLE

3. *Luteal phase.* This is the phase during which PMS occurs. After the egg has been released, what is left of the
follicle that housed it becomes a functioning gland called
the corpus luteum. This Latin term means "yellow body"
and refers to the yellow pigment of the lutein it has absorbed in the process of changing from follicle to gland.
The corpus luteum produces progesterone and small
amounts of estrogen during the next ten to fourteen days.
This progesterone surge is what causes a raised basal body
temperature, which is one way to document that ovulation
has occurred. It also maintains the thickened lining of the
uterus and its new blood supply. If in about fourteen days a
pregnancy has not occurred, the corpus luteum ceases to
function.

4. *Menstruation.* As the corpus luteum produces less progesterone and finally stops, the endometrium responds by
releasing chemicals called prostaglandins just before the
menstrual period begins, and for some women, into the
first few days of it. The result is uterine cramping, and for
some people, nausea, vomiting, and backache, all of which
are known as dysmenorrhea. Prostaglandins may also play a
role in PMS. Since the levels of estrogen and progesterone
have now dropped dramatically, the endometrium stops
growing, and the tiny arteries that formed to feed the new
tissue close off. Without oxygen and nutrients from the
blood supply to feed them, cells in the endometrium and
the arteries themselves begin dying and breaking up. As
they break up, the arteries begin to bleed again, and this
blood along with the sloughed-off cells of the endometrium
appears as menstrual discharge. Menstrual bleeding lasts
from three to seven days in most women and consists of
between four to twelve teaspoonfuls of blood.

As the brain senses lowered estrogen levels that result

from menstruation, it signals the hypothalamus to begin a new cycle.

THEORETICAL CAUSES OF PMS

While there doesn't seem to be a single cause of PMS, there are plenty of theories. For the most part, they relate to the hormone activity from ovulation to the beginning of the menstrual period—the last two weeks of the cycle—or to the effects of diet and exercise on hormone production. While these theories form the basis for many of the treatments available now, keep in mind that they remain theories. None of them provides the whole answer to relief from PMS for everyone. Finding a personalized approach to PMS will require that you understand your symptoms thoroughly so that you and your physician choose only the parts of these theories and the treatments they suggest that address your symptoms. The descriptions here include arguments for and against each theory.

Theory 1: The Hormone Deficiency/Hormone Excess Theory. There are three parts to this theory. The first states that women with PMS have a *progesterone deficiency* during the luteal phase of their cycles that causes PMS symptoms. But recent studies have shown that women who have a documented luteal phase progesterone deficiency have no greater PMS symptoms than those who don't. This theory seems to have been further debunked by studies in recent years to determine the effectiveness of progesterone supplementation in treating PMS symptoms, including a landmark study reported in a July 1991 edition of the *Journal of the American Medical Association*. The studies show no difference between the effects of a placebo and progesterone supplements on PMS symptoms. However, in the United States progesterone supplementation is one of the most commonly prescribed treatments for PMS, and anecdotal evidence shows that some women see some improvement when they use progesterone supplementation.

The second part of this theory states that PMS symptoms may be caused by an *excess of estrogen,* which occurs during ovulation, when estrogen amounts can increase to as much as six times the amount present during other times of the cycle. The counterargument to this theory holds that if excess estrogen production were to blame, the most severe PMS symptoms would occur during ovulation, *not* nearer the beginning of the menstrual period, as is the case for most women. A very few women do have their most severe symptoms during ovulation, but more commonly, women have a feeling of well-being then. And some studies have shown that estrogen may actually have an antidepressant effect.

The third part of this theory is the opposite of the first part. It states that PMS symptoms are caused by *exposure to increased progesterone.* Studies have shown that some women experience PMS types of symptoms when they are given natural or synthetic progesterone supplements during the late follicular phase (just before ovulation). Even some women who have gone through menopause develop PMS-like symptoms when they take an estrogen replacement product that contains progesterone.

Theory 2: The Excess Prostaglandins Theory. Some investigators believe that a number of PMS symptoms occur because of an increase in prostaglandins during the luteal phase of the menstrual cycle—the time between ovulation and menstruation. They have shown that because of the decrease in progesterone just before menstruation begins, the endometrium releases the chemicals called prostaglandins, which are known to alter smooth muscle tone, immune function, and the brain's neurotransmitter metabolism. These changes may have a role in the moodiness some women experience with PMS.

Theory 3: The Vitamin B_6 Deficiency Theory. No objective evidence shows a vitamin B_6 deficiency in women with PMS that coincides with their menstrual cycles, and studies on the effects of taking B_6 supplements have shown varying results. In the studies in which B_6 was proved helpful, though, the vitamin improved subjects' mood over *both* phases of the cycle, indicating that subjects may have been generally deficient in vitamin B_6. Wide-ranging studies have not been done on the specific effects of nutritional deficiencies on PMS, but anecdotal evidence shows that for many women, better nutrition means they feel better during their PMS times. Many nonmedical treatments, including taking vitamins, minerals, herbs, amino acids, dietary fiber, and essential fatty acids, are based on the same thinking as this theory: that a deficiency in one or more of these substances is a primary cause of PMS symptoms; when no deficiency exists, these substances can help improve a woman's general health enough that she feels better all month, including her PMS times.

Theory 4: The Exposure/Withdrawal Beta-Endorphin Theory. Recent evidence suggests that beta-endorphins, the "feel-good" hormones or opiates produced in your hypothalamus, are profoundly affected by estrogen and progesterone levels in your body. Studies on primates whose menstrual cycles and PMS behaviors mimic those of humans have shown that their beta-endorphin levels rise through the mid- to late-follicular phase and peak during the mid-luteal phase. At menstruation, when hormone output is at its lowest level, beta-endorphin concentrations in the blood are all but undetectable. Withdrawal from the high opiate levels may be linked to irritability, aggressive behavior, irregular body temperature, sleep disturbance, headaches, and diarrhea. The intensity of the symptoms seems to have a lot to do with the degree and duration of exposure to high levels of opiates and with how rapidly the levels fall. Many of these mood and behavioral changes have been duplicated in human volunteers.

Increased exercise as a treatment for PMS is based on this theory. Strenuous, sustained exercise produces beta-endorphins, or the "runner's high." The theory holds that by exercising regularly, a woman can counteract the natural drop in beta-endorphins during her cycle, avoiding some mood swings. No studies have proved this, but many women report they feel better and their PMS symptoms seem less bothersome when they undertake regular exercise programs.

Practicing yoga helps some women reduce PMS symptoms, even though beta-endorphins are usually associated with aerobic exercise. Acupuncture and acupressure, which seek to rechannel the body's flow of electrical energy to relieve PMS symptoms, may also relate to this theory.

Theory 5: The Changing Circadian Rhythm Theory. Changing circadian rhythms (the biological clock by which the body's timing is set) across the menstrual cycle may be responsible for PMS symptoms in some women in much the same way that jet lag affects some people. Researchers have found striking similarities between travelers with jet lag and women with PMS. They share transitory symptoms, lasting two to seven days for the most part, including nocturnal sleep disturbance and daytime sleepiness, mood changes, difficulty concentrating on tasks, appetite changes, and nausea. Animal studies have shown that the hormones that govern menstrual cycles affect biological rhythms. For example, sleep activity patterns are affected by estrogen during the estrous cycle of hamsters. Similar changes have been seen in monkeys, and some researchers believe these relate as well to humans. Consequently, getting more sleep during premenstrual times is helpful to some women.

Five more theories address a limited number of PMS symptoms:

The Low-Grade Infection Theory. Some physicians believe that a low-grade infection within the genital tract can be the cause of some physical PMS symptoms like fatigue, backaches, and the tendency toward the appearance of cystitis symptoms. Their theory is based on the fact that some women show improvement in PMS symptoms when they are given the antibiotic doxycycline.

The Systemic Yeast Infection Theory. This theory is also the result of noting the effects of a treatment for something other than PMS. Some women treated with nystatin, which is active against yeast and other fungi, showed improvement of several physical PMS symptoms, but not of depression.

The Excess Prolactin Theory. Prolactin is the hormone that helps produce breast milk, and certain studies during the last six or eight years have centered on its role in breast-related PMS symptoms like pain and swelling. They have shown that prolactin is apparently a significant factor in PMS-related breast discomfort. Some medical treatments address these breast-only symptoms.

Other theories only recently in favor have been generally discredited. It's helpful to know about those, too, when you are considering what treatment will work for you.

The Hypoglycemia Theory. At one time it was thought that hypoglycemia (low blood sugar caused by abnormal function of the pancreas) was a contributing factor in PMS because for some women hypoglycemialike symptoms appeared during the late luteal phase. But oral glucose tolerance tests, which are used to diagnose hypoglycemia, have failed to show any significant differences in oral glucose tolerance or insulin secretion at different phases of the menstrual cycle.

The Allergic-to-Your-Own-Hormones Theory. This theory was espoused for a while several years ago, and it gained a little support when some studies showed that women with PMS generally have a higher than normal incidence of allergic symptoms in their families. Not enough evidence has been found to support this hypothesis seriously, but this theory, along with the results of a few more recent studies, is the reason drug companies include antihistamines in over-the-counter PMS preparations.

LIFE PHASES

Even though the exact way hormones affect PMS remains poorly understood, it is clear that PMS is intimately linked to the activity of the hypothalamus, pituitary, and ovaries and the substances they produce. And that relationship helps define *when* PMS is most likely to have an effect on you during different phases of your life.

Prepuberty and Puberty. PMS symptoms have been documented in some girls before the beginning of their first periods. This is probably due to the sporadic production of estrogen by ovarian follicles that sometimes occurs. But it is much more typical for PMS not to occur until ovarian function is in full swing, after menarche. And while some adolescents report intense PMS symptoms, it is not widespread in this age-group.

Twenties and Thirties. If women didn't have PMS in their teens, they probably won't in their twenties. They may find, however, that some symptoms appear in their late twenties and slowly increase or intensify during their thirties. Some will find that taking birth control pills produces PMS or intensifies symptoms. For others who have had PMS all along, there may be some relief during pregnancy, when the cyclic production of hormones stops. When it resumes after the birth of a baby or even after a miscarriage or abortion, those who've never had PMS may find they're experiencing symptoms.

It's important to note for this age-group, as well as for the later age-group, that cyclic *menstruation or ovulation is not itself a prerequisite for PMS*. All it takes is hormone production to produce the symptoms. That's why if, like millions of other women in the United States, you decide to have a tubal ligation, any PMS symptoms you had before will still be around after the surgery.

Forties and Fifties. While you may see changes in the length of your menstrual cycle during your forties, it doesn't mean you'll necessarily see a lessening in PMS symptoms. But if you haven't had serious PMS by now, it's not likely to appear, since hormone production may be waning. It's normal for many women in their forties to miss a period occasionally or to have some anovulatory cycles (during which no ovulation takes place), but as long as hormone production is intact, PMS symptoms are likely to be too. Some women find it especially frustrating to deal with irregular periods *and* with unpredictable PMS symptoms.

The average age for menopause in this country is fifty-one to fifty-two years, and it is this cessation of cyclic hormonal activity that stops PMS. However, it's important to note that, like a tubal ligation, a premenopause hysterectomy that leaves the ovaries intact will do nothing for your PMS. PMS symptoms have been reported in some women whose hysterectomies left the tiniest bit of ovarian tissue behind. Some women also find they have occasional PMS days within the first year after menopause for the same reason some girls have PMS occasionally before menarche: sporadic estrogen production by ovarian follicles.

DO YOU HAVE PMS?

If you are feeling confused and depressed about your symptoms, it may be hard to initiate the process of identifying the problems you're having. Give yourself some time to read and mull over the information in this book, and then try to take action one step at a time. Successful PMS diagnosis and treatment happen just that way—one small step at a time.

In this chapter you will find hints on how to chart your symptoms to get the information you need, how to select the best health care provider for you, and what to expect in an initial visit with the health care provider you choose.

CHARTING YOUR SYMPTOMS

As of this writing, there is no blood test, no physical exam, no psychological testing that, used alone, can tell you if what you're experiencing is PMS. The only way to diagnose your PMS is for *you* to keep a chart of your symptoms and of the times they occur in your menstrual cycle during two or three cycles.

That is not to say that you shouldn't consult a health

care provider. But it is to say that when you do, whether you see your own gynecologist or someone at a PMS clinic, your diagnosis and treatment should center on the symptom chart you develop and what that chart shows.

The point of charting is:

—to define your symptoms clearly

—to see when your symptoms start and stop

—to see which symptoms occur during which part of the cycle

One way to chart symptoms is to use a graph format, with a list of symptoms running down the left side and with days of the month running across the top. Choose symbols to represent whether the symptom is nonexistent, mild, moderate, or severe. Each day mark the appropriate squares beneath the day of the month with the symbol that describes how you feel. Circle the days of menstruation and ovulation. If you can't tell when you ovulate (usually the midpoint of your cycle, around Day 13 to 15; some women feel a little pain or cramping in their lower abdomens or see heavier vaginal mucus discharge), you might want to take your temperature for a couple of months to find out. To do so, you need a basal body temperature thermometer from a pharmacy. Instructions will come with it, but all you do is put the thermometer in your mouth for five minutes each morning before you get out of bed. Your temperature should rise a degree or two when you ovulate (as explained in Chapter 2) and then fall twenty-four to forty-eight hours afterward.

Your chart might look like this:

0 = none   m = mild   M = moderate   S = severe

	1	2	3	4	5	6	7	8	9	10	11	12	13	14	15	16	17	18	19	20	21	22	23	24	25	26	27	28	29	30
Loss of emotional control																														
Anxiety																														
Decreased concentration																														
Depression																														
Nightmares																														
Mood swings																														
Headaches, migraines																														
Joint and muscle aches																														
Backaches																														
Food cravings																														
Decreased alcohol tolerance																														

	1	2	3	4	5	6	7	8	9	10	11	12	13	14	15	16	17	18	19	20	21	22	23	24	25	26	27	28	29	30
Clumsiness																														
Changes in sex drive																														
Constipation, diarrhea																														
Shakiness, dizziness																														
Cystitis, urethritis																														
Abdominal bloating																														
Skin problems																														
Breast tenderness																														

H = headache;   B = bloated;   I = irritable;   P =period, etc.

	April	May	June
1			
2			H
3		H&B	B
4		H&B	B
5	H&B	H&I	H&I
6	H&B	H	P
7	H&I	I	P
8	H&I	P	P
9	H	P	P
10	P	P	
11	P	P	
12	P		
13	P		

To set up a chart that runs for several months, write the month at the top and the days of the month down the left side. Fill in symptoms on the days they occur. This chart helps you see a recurring pattern, month to month.

In addition to a symptoms chart, you should keep a brief journal that lists what you eat, whether you exercise, and how you feel—emotionally and physically—each day. Not only will your journal help you collect clues to the ways food and exercise affect you, but the information will also help you zero in on life-style changes you may need to make.

You can also chart symptoms on your computer. There is a software program called PMS Analysis for IBM compatible and Apple II series computers that accomplishes the same task as the charts above. It also produces a personalized report with recommended life-style changes to help you with the particular symptom patterns your chart shows you have.

If all this sounds like a lot of work, most women report it isn't really. Once you get started, charting should take just a few minutes a day, and the rewards you'll reap in understanding your cycle and how PMS symptoms relate to it can be tremendous.

GETTING MEDICAL HELP

When you decide to see someone about your symptoms, give some thought to what kind of care giver you should see. As explained in Chapter 1, PMS crosses the boundaries between disciplines by being a biobehavioral condition, one that involves psychological as well as physical systems. The most effective care giver will be a person who can work with both aspects of PMS.

Keep in mind that PMS is not a subject that is taught in medical schools, although some schools may have a lecture or two on the topic. While some gynecologists may be sensitive to PMS as a real condition as opposed to one that's "all in your head," unless they have taken on the diagnosis and treatment of PMS as a special interest and have engaged in a great deal of self-education, they may not be up on the latest developments in treatment. And while some psychologists may understand the dynamics of what happens in your relationships during your PMS time, they are probably not trained to deal with the physical realities of PMS.

You may find just the middle ground you need at a PMS clinic. At reputable clinics (see the Resource List in the back of this book), you will find professionals trained in all the aspects of PMS who either work with a physician on staff or would work with your physician if need be. But be discerning in whom you choose to see: PMS has been the topic of scores of media reports during the last ten years, so beware of unqualified personnel and clinics that may be trying to cash in on a trend.

As you look for a PMS expert, you can check with:

—your own gynecologist for his or her expertise in PMS

—your own gynecologist or your family doctor for his or her recommendation of a PMS expert

—your state health department

—a women's health center, if there is one, associated with your local hospital

—the Resource List at the end of this book

—the yellow pages of the telephone book for a PMS clinic near you

How to know who will be right for you? You are looking for a health care provider who is willing to study your symptoms and to develop an individualized treatment program for you. Someone who:

—doesn't generalize ("All women benefit from hormone supplementation.")

—doesn't minimize ("Your symptoms don't sound that bad.")

—believes in your ability to report symptoms accurately

THE CONSULTATION

No matter what kind of health care provider you are considering, the first step is to schedule a consultation *before* your first "real" appointment. A consultation is a clothes-on, face-to-face conversation during which you can find out about the individual's knowledge of and approach to PMS. You may be talking to a physician, a physician's assistant, or a nurse practitioner, but be sure that at least a part of your consultation is with the person you would be working with. Be prepared to pay an office visit fee for the professional's time, although some clinics and physicians don't charge or charge a lesser fee for consultations.

Bring your completed chart and journal to the consultation. With them, you will be able to show clearly a record of your menstrual periods, their duration, your ovulation times, and how your symptoms coincide with each of these. Ask the health care provider to look them over. While no one wants to be asked to make a snap decision, you should be able to get an opinion on whether it appears you have PMS or not.

Don't be discouraged if the physician agrees you probably have PMS and throws up his or her hands, saying that there's no cure, that you just have to learn to live with it. All that means is that this doctor is not familiar enough with PMS to work with you. While research has not ferreted out a *single* cause and does not point to a *single* miracle cure for PMS, still, there are more than fifty different treatments for it (many of which are discussed in the following chapters), and *all* of them work to some degree for some women. So if the health care provider you are consulting with tells you to "learn to live with it," find a new health care provider.

If you get a more positive response, then you will need to question that person further to understand his or her approach to PMS. Some things you should ask:

—How many PMS patients does the health care provider see? Whether you go to a PMS clinic or a private physician, this is a good question to help you get an idea of how much experience lies behind the treatment program. Your treatment will be different if you are the first PMS patient this provider has seen or the hundredth.

—Would the health care provider feel comfortable referring you elsewhere? What if, in a diligent search for answers about your PMS, a physical problem of some sort appears? What if you need some kind of medication that this person is unprepared or unqualified to dispense? You will want to know if there are physicians on staff who can handle any potential situation or if certain patients are referred to other physicians.

—What is his or her approach to PMS? You are looking for an answer that lets you know that you and your needs will be the center of the treatment. Flexibility and individual focus are the keys to getting that kind of help.

—Is he or she prepared to treat your PMS as a biobehavioral condition? Since PMS symptoms can be both psychological and physical, it's important that treatment addresses both aspects. Asking exactly how this care giver treats each of these will help you make a decision.

—How does this clinic or individual react to ideas from informed patients? The most successful treatment of PMS requires a partnership between care giver and patient.

—How many office visits are needed, and how are they billed? Since you are looking for an individualized program, the frequency of visits may vary according to whom you see. Sometime during your first visit or two to a physician or a clinic, you need to hear a detailed explanation of how the program works. It's also a good idea to check with your insurance company to see if PMS treatment is routinely covered and to ask the health care provider what his or her experience has been with insurance coverage.

—What support services are available through this office? Education and peer support groups are helpful for most women. It's convenient if these are provided in one place. If not, the health care provider should be able to tell you how and when you can find these services through another office or clinic.

THE FIRST VISIT

When you arrive for the first visit, the person or assistant you are seeing should take a complete history from you. This process will be simpler if you have your chart and journal with you. Questions care givers should ask:

—What symptoms (psychological and physical) do you have that lead you to believe you have PMS?

—Which is the biggest problem for you?

—When do the symptoms start and end in relation to your menstrual cycle?

—When did you first realize your symptoms were cyclical? Did you discover this? If not, who pointed it out to you?

—How do your symptoms affect your relationships with family, friends, coworkers? Do they interfere with your optimum functioning?

—Have your symptoms increased, decreased, or stayed the same over time?

—When did your symptoms first begin?

You should also be asked about your medical history, including such questions as:

—Have you taken or are you taking oral contraceptives? How do/did they affect your symptoms?

—Have you experienced toxemia of pregnancy, postpartum depression, miscarriage, abortion, tubal ligation, hysterectomy? How did these affect your symptoms?

—How many pregnancies have you had? Did you notice symptoms appearing or disappearing during or after these?

—Do you think or know your mother, sister(s), or daughter(s) had or have PMS?

Specific questions about your menstrual cycle should be part of the medical history. Unless you have already done some charting, you may not know all the answers to these at your first visit.

—How long is your menstrual cycle? Count the first day of your period as Day 1. The length of your cycle is the total number of days until the first day of your next period.

—When in this cycle do your symptoms go away?

—How do you feel when your period begins? When it ends?

—Do you have a symptom-free time during your cycle?

—Does your sex drive change during your cycle?

Several life-style habits have been seen to contribute to PMS, so you should be questioned about your current diet and exercise habits as well as stress levels in your life. Care givers may simply ask about your intake of things like sugar, caffeine, vitamins, and highly refined foods, along with how many times a week you exercise and what kind of exercise you do. Or if you haven't already done so, they may have you go home and chart what you do eat each day and note down each day's exercise and how you feel.

A health care provider who is sensitive to PMS should also take into account what has been happening in your life in the last year or so. For example, if you have just moved to a new house with a mortgage a tick over what you think fits comfortably into your budget, if you have received an award for outstanding performance at work, and if your six-year-old has just started first grade, that can tell a practitioner that you may be under enough stress to need all the coaching you can get about taking care of yourself.

Even if you haven't had any emotional big events recently, there is normal daily stress to consider too. Your doctor or PMS counselor should ask you about what's happening with work, with your partner, and with your family, about what's happening now *inside* you, where your self-esteem and your spirit live, that may be adding to the stress in your life.

On top of that, she or he should find out from you how stress specifically affects your body. Do you feel it in rock-hard muscles in your shoulders and neck? Do you invariably get a headache over your eyes when the going gets tough? Is it your aching lower back or the knot in your stomach that tells you it's been a rough day?

A start-up exam will also include some kind of psychiatric examination administered during the first part, or follicular phase, of your cycle. This is usually in the form of a questionnaire you fill out or an interview with a qualified person like a psychologist or a counselor. It is important that this be done during the follicular phase of your cycle, when you do not have the symptoms that concern you, so that you and your physician can discern if there is an underlying psychiatric problem. If there is, you may be able to see that PMS intensifies the problem; if there is not, you can more clearly attribute your psychological symptoms to PMS. Some clinics may do a similar evaluation during the week or so before your period, when your symptoms are likely to be at their peak, to define their effect further.

Most physicians will also want to do a pelvic exam and Pap smear, draw blood for a blood count and chemistry screen, and ask for a urine sample. While none of these will tell your doctor if you *do* have PMS, these exams may help you and the physician determine what your symptoms *are not*.

WHAT ELSE COULD YOUR
SYMPTOMS MEAN?

It's not uncommon for PMS to be misdiagnosed partly because it can show up in almost any body system (as in migraines, eye problems, and chronic conditions like asthma that worsen premenstrually) and partly because some health care providers are not familiar enough with it. On the other hand, it is possible to dismiss certain symptoms as PMS when they can indicate another condition. You can help your health care provider sort out what is PMS and what isn't by knowing about some of the conditions that look like it.

Chronic Epstein-Barr Virus. CEBV is an incurable illness that results from the activation of a type of herpes virus (called EBV) which is present in nearly all humans, often from birth. This virus may live benignly in the body, it can trigger mononucleosis, or it can flourish to become CEBV. Many of the symptoms of CEBV and PMS overlap, including extreme lassitude, anxiety, depression, difficulty concentrating, joint pain, and confusion. No link has been found between the two disorders, but there are a few important differences:

—Unlike PMS, CEBV occurs suddenly. PMS tends to worsen slowly over time. CEBV may begin as a severe cold or flu that never goes away.

—Symptoms of CEBV do not disappear at certain times, as do PMS symptoms.

—CEBV can be totally disabling, whereas women can usually work around PMS.

—Exercise can make CEBV worse, whereas it often helps women with PMS.

There is a blood test to discern levels of antibodies to EBV, which are often high if a person has CEBV. But testing methods are still crude and unreliable, with 30 percent of people who have CEBV symptoms testing normal for EBV antibodies. The most reliable way to tell if what you have is PMS or CEBV is to chart your symptoms. If they are cyclical, they are most likely not CEBV.

Panic Disorders. Panic attacks and acute anxiety are often reported as symptoms of PMS. But those alone don't mean you have a panic disorder. People with panic disorders have paralyzing, debilitating conditions that limit their lives and, in severe cases, immobilize them completely. For most of them, there will be panic attacks (episodes of extreme anxiety manifested by a pounding heart, shortness of breath, chest pain, headache, dizziness, trembling), which will occur with increasing frequency and magnitude over time.

Even if you do have panic attacks, the key to being sure whether or not they are caused by PMS is to chart your symptoms. If the attacks are cyclical, they are probably not a panic disorder.

Dysmenorrhea. This is pelvic pain or menstrual cramping that generally begins a day before your period and ends sometime during or at the end of the flow. Dysmenorrhea occurs separately from PMS: You may have one and not the other, or you may have both. But since dysmenorrhea is not a condition that exists cyclically in the two weeks between ovulation and menstruation, it is not part of PMS and should be treated separately.

Endometriosis. This painful condition is marked by heavy bleeding and cramping during periods. As with dysmenorrhea, endometrial pain is sometimes mistaken for PMS. Endometriosis is caused by cells from the endometrium (lining of the uterus) growing elsewhere throughout the pelvic cavity, including the outside of the uterus, the ovaries, uterine ligaments, vagina, and cervix, and in some cases in other parts of the body. These implants of endometrial cells bleed during menstruation in response to hormone levels in the body. While symptoms of endometriosis will be cyclical because they center on the menstrual period, implants can be revealed by internal exams, including laparoscopy to view the inside of the pelvic cavity with special instruments inserted through a tiny incision near the navel. Heavy periods and cramping, whether they are ultimately shown to be endometriosis or not, have nothing to do with PMS.

Depressive Disorders. Depression is part of PMS for many women, but ongoing, unremitting depression is not. Some depressive disorders for which PMS has been mistaken are *cyclothymic disorder,* characterized by numerous episodes of depression over a period of at least two years; *dysthymic disorder,* characterized by a chronic mood disturbance of about two years' duration along with a loss of interest in most activities; and *major depressive episode,* which is marked by a loss of interest or pleasure in all activities, along with persistent depression, hopelessness, sadness, and/or irritability.

Once again the primary way to tell the difference between these and PMS lies in charting symptoms and discerning cyclical changes in mood.

Thyroid Disease. Symptoms resulting from hyperthyroidism often resemble those of PMS—for example, increased nervousness or emotional instability. However, a blood test can tell you if you have a problem with your thyroid; your charts can tell you if your symptoms are cyclical.

Diabetes. Many women with PMS are extremely thirsty or have eating binges premenstrually. People with diabetes do, too, but not in a cyclical manner. Urine and blood tests can tell you if you have diabetes.

Hypoglycemia. PMS and hypoglycemia share many symptoms, including anxiety, nervousness, weakness, fatigue, headache, restlessness, difficulty with speech and thinking, agitation, prolonged sleep, and temper outbursts.

If you have hypoglycemia, charting symptoms with regard to eating *and* your menstrual cycle will show that your symptoms are not limited to the luteal phase of your cycle.

By now it should be clear that one of the primary characteristics of PMS is that it is cyclical and that if you weren't convinced before, it is *absolutely necessary* that you chart your symptoms if you want to gain control over them. It's also important to note that if you already know you have any of the conditions listed here, PMS may make their symptoms worse during the luteal phase of your cycle.

SUPPORT GROUPS AND COUNSELING

Once you have figured out that your symptoms are PMS, then education and support are vital to you and should be the first concern of an experienced health care provider. A good program can help you improve your own coping mechanisms, learn how to reduce stress, and strengthen and use effectively the support systems you already have. Women who have participated in qualified ongoing PMS support groups report comfort in knowing they are not alone in their struggle to gain control over their PMS. They say that the group experience validates their symptoms and their efforts to manage them. In addition, the groups offer education about the physical process that produces PMS, a better understanding of individual needs, and an opportunity to share information about techniques that work. Perhaps most important, they also offer recognition that you are not just crazy.

Some options you may want to consider:

—brief couple or family therapy with a qualified psychologist or PMS counselor. This educates not only you but your family about the cyclic nature of PMS symptoms and helps all of you learn about coping and aiding you in dealing with the symptoms.

—group therapy, particularly through a PMS center or clinic. Some clinics have groups that meet for a set period of time and offer a special curriculum for dealing with aspects of PMS, like using symptom charts to manage symptoms, learning stress reduction techniques, improving patterns of communication, organizing a nutrition and fitness program, restructuring negative views of oneself to avoid depression, etc.

As you look for a support group, there are three more considerations to help you choose. Probably the key issue in your feeling comfortable in a group is trust. If you don't feel safe exploring your feelings, no matter how well run the group may be, it won't help you. One way to develop that trust and a feeling of safety is for you to ascertain ahead of time that the group's proceedings are confidential. If you want to know, ask the leader or facilitator what her policy is.

That brings you to the second factor: Who will lead the group? A skilled facilitator, experienced and knowledgeable about the issues surrounding PMS, is the ideal person. Without focus and leadership, groups tend to wander during discussions, attendance may flag, and the safety net of confidentiality may disappear. Ask about the qualifications of the facilitator and how she handles group discussions before you join. Keep in mind, too, that if you attend a group session and you just don't like the facilitator, it is your prerogative to change groups. Think of the process of selecting a group as similar to that of finding a good therapist or counselor; all the degrees and experience in the world don't matter if you don't have a good personality fit.

The facilitator's viewpoint should have a strong effect, too, on the third factor: the atmosphere of the meetings. There are many valid ways to approach dealing with PMS, and the only requirement is that the approach used is a positive one. A "misery loves company" tone will not help.

FOUR

GAIN CONTROL BY CHANGING YOUR LIFE-STYLE

Once you are sure your symptoms are PMS, the first, and for many women the best, treatment should be the simplest. After education and support the next step for you to take is to look into changing your life-style.

As with most of the research that has to do with PMS, studies on the effects of dietary changes and increased exercise show mixed results, but that's not necessarily bad. While research does say that these changes don't work for everyone, it also says that they *do* work for many women. And these kinds of changes produce the plus of having only positive side effects: a generally healthier you.

DIETARY CHANGES

If you've checked your local library or bookstore lately for books on PMS, you may have noticed plenty of "PMS diets." For the most part these diets are based on a few simple principles:

1. *Restricting caffeine.* While coffee, tea, and cola drinks don't cause PMS, caffeine intake has been linked with more severe premenstrual symptoms, from mood swings and anxiety to breast tenderness and bloatedness. In addition, caffeine itself can cause irritability, insomnia, and gastrointestinal distress at any time, so it is only sensible to limit its intake during the time when you may be more subject to those anyway. If you usually drink more than about four cups of coffee a day, stopping all at once can cause caffeine-withdrawal headaches. Try cutting back by a half cup a day at first and substituting a decaffeinated beverage or herb tea.

2. *Limiting salt.* Many PMS symptoms, like weight gain, joint pain, and headache, are associated with fluid retention. And while studies have shown that those symptoms are caused in most women by the *shifting* of fluid rather than by *additional* fluid, still, overconsumption of salt (typical of most Americans, according to the American Cancer Society guidelines) can lead to temporary weight gain.

You can reduce your salt intake by removing the salt shaker from your table. If you really like to season your food with salt, try a potassium-based salt substitute, or add a few grains of sea salt to an herb mixture. You can also try limiting high-salt foods to one every three days or so. Some high-salt foods to moderate your intake of are:

—most convenience foods, like frozen dinners and frozen pizza

—preserved or smoked meats, like salami, ham, pastrami, bacon, hot dogs, sausage, corned beef

—bouillon cubes, instant soups, canned soups (except the salt-free variety)

—Worcestershire, soy, and steak sauce; gravy mixes

—potato chips and other chips

—food in brine, like relish, pickles, olives

—canned fish, like anchovies, tuna, salmon, sardines, and caviar

—instant foods, like cereals and potatoes; packaged drink mixes, like hot chocolate

—salty seasonings, like garlic salt, onion salt, MSG, mustard, ketchup, prepared horseradish

3. *Cutting back on sweets, including chocolate.* Although you may crave chocolate, especially during PMS times, remember it is a concentrated source of sugar *and* caffeine. Large quantities of sugar seem to make worse some premenstrual symptoms like depression and fatigue, and some nutritionists believe that too much of either sugar or chocolate can deplete the body's B complex vitamins, which you need to lessen fatigue. For most women, giving in to a sugar or chocolate craving only perpetuates itself: You'll most likely just feel like eating more. Try eating something sour or bitter, like one pickle, when you're craving sugar; for some people it stops a sweets binge. Even though pickles are salty, and you may also be trying to avoid salt, moderation rather than exclusion is the rule. If you really crave something sweet, substitute unsweetened apple juice or a more concentrated sweetener like honey or maple syrup for sugar. The apple juice allows you to avoid sugar altogether, and you need much less honey or syrup than sugar to get that sweet taste. Carob, a member of the legume family that is high in calcium, is a reasonable substitute for chocolate and won't cause the kinds of mood swings chocolate does in some people. You can get carob at a health food store in chunk form for baking, powdered for drinks, and as part of some candies and cookies. But read the label before you buy; carob products can be just as high in sugar as chocolate products.

If you're cooking or baking, you can usually cut the amount of sugar called for by one-third to one-half without affecting the recipe. And in case you do decide to have a dessert or sweet during your PMS time, try not to do it often. Having dessert once in two or three days is far better than having it after two meals in one day.

4. *Cutting down on alcohol.* Many women who usually have no problem with alcohol find they do during their PMS times. You may find that you have less tolerance for alcohol (perhaps one drink has the effect of two) or that alcohol only intensifies symptoms like irritability, anxiety, and headache. See if you can do without it during your PMS times, or substitute light (low-alcohol) wine or beer.

5. *Eating less, but more often.* While hypoglycemia (low blood sugar caused by abnormal function of the pancreas) and PMS are different things, and while links between the two remain to be proved, some women report that following a basic hypoglycemia diet all month long helps their PMS symptoms. A hypoglycemia diet is one that includes protein and complex carbohydrates but that is low in simple carbohydrates like refined sugar and is moderate in fats. It consists of five or six *small* meals a day, which offer a constant supply of nutrients to your body to keep your blood sugar at a more constant level. A rule of thumb is never to go more than three hours during the day without a small meal or snack.

6. *Adding complex carbohydrates.* At least one study has shown that women with PMS who ate a carbohydrate-rich diet (including whole grain bread, rice, pasta, and potatoes) were less depressed and irritable and more mentally alert. This may be because carbohydrates stimulate the brain to produce more of the neurotransmitter serotonin, which helps ease depression and tension. Adding foods like those mentioned above, along with more fruits and vegetables, may help you. If you're watching your weight, try low-fat additions like popcorn, rice cakes, animal crackers, or even angel food cake. Eating more carbohydrates does not mean you have to go for the ice cream, cookies, and other high-fat, high-sugar foods.

FOODS THAT SEEM TO HELP

There is no "perfect food" that will erase your PMS symptoms, but there are a few that many women find help them moderate or avoid PMS symptoms. Most provide nutrients you need anyway. Many nutritionists believe it's best to get these nutrients from foods rather than supplements and that fresh rather than cooked foods supply more of the nutrients you're looking for. Others believe supplements can be just as helpful. Chapter 6 offers a list of vitamin and food supplements you might find useful.

Here are some foods you can add and what they can do for you:

—leafy green vegetables, liver, legumes, whole grains, nuts: for B complex vitamins to combat fatigue and irritability

—avocados, whole grain cereals, wheat germ, soybeans, bananas, green peppers: for vitamin B_6 to decrease irritability, fatigue, mood swings, and food cravings and possibly to reduce headache and breast swelling

—broccoli, turnip greens, safflower oil: for vitamin E to relieve breast tenderness

—spinach, cabbage, seeds, nuts, and shellfish: for magnesium to help control sugar cravings, mood swings, and nervous tension

Another simple change that women often overlook is to drink eight glasses of water a day, not including coffee, soda, or tea. Contrary to how it may seem, drinking *more* water rather than *less* can help relieve your bloated feeling, because water has a cleansing effect that helps your whole digestive system work better. A glass of water can help you stay away from the coffeepot or the candy machine at work too. If you don't drink that much water now, you may have to work up to it, both for the sake of your sanity as you set out to make more than one change and for the sake of your bladder, which may not be used to processing such quantities.

PLANNING AHEAD

As you work to incorporate these changes into your diet, a couple of key principles will help you. Perhaps the most important one is: *Plan ahead.* If you know you're going to have a crazy day running from meeting to meeting or doing errands with a two-year-old, bring a snack for yourself. Pack three or four crackers with a teaspoonful of peanut butter on each, an apple with an ounce of cheese, or a half sandwich. Any of these will see you through better than another cup of coffee or a candy bar. But you have to plan ahead in order to have the food you need when you need it.

Another is: *Don't skip meals.* If you feel bloated, for example, skipping a meal won't help, but it will set you up for overeating when you get so hungry you can't control your impulse to eat. And the lowered blood sugar you may experience after skipping a meal could set you up for an angry outburst, depression, or an anxiety attack.

Many experts say that in order to get the full benefit from these healthy habits, you must maintain them through the whole month. But it wouldn't hurt to be particularly vigilant during the two weeks before your period.

As you are planning your meals and snacks, remember that a balanced meal includes:

—complex carbohydrates, like potatoes, rice, noodles, corn, beans, peas, breads. Whole grains, rather than processed, bleached grains, offer more B vitamins and fiber.

—protein, like chicken, fish, beef, veal, lamb, cheese. Some people like to cut back on red meat during their PMS times, primarily because of the estrogen that's injected into many cattle, although there have been no definitive studies to show the effects of estrogen in beef on PMS symptoms. But if it makes you feel better, do it, and replace it with another protein.

—vegetables, with the emphasis on raw to get the maximum nutrients.

—fruits. Eat three a day: an orange for vitamin C, an apple with skin for fiber, and one other favorite.

—milk or yogurt, six ounces a day minimum. Some
people also feel better eating fewer dairy products on
their PMS days. If you do, get calcium from another
food source, like sardines or salmon with bones.

Most conventional health care providers agree that these
dietary changes make the most sense and help many
women. However, always be aware of what works best for
you; you are the final authority on your body.

IMPORTANCE OF EXERCISE

In the late 1970s and early 1980s aerobic exercise was first
scientifically recognized as having a positive psychological
effect. One study showed that psychiatric patients who engaged in a regular program of running were less depressed;
another showed that during prolonged aerobic exercise the
brain produced more beta-endorphins, creating the runner's high. Because both depression and a lack of beta-
endorphins have been linked with PMS, the good effects of
exercise is great news for women.

Since those first studies, others have shown that regular
exercise, whether an energetic walking program or an aerobics class, can help relieve the severity of some PMS symptoms. Some women report they have less breast tenderness,
fluid retention, and bloatedness when they work out during
their PMS times. And it just makes sense that having a
physical outlet for pent-up energy will help.

Many women think of exercise as a preventive measure.
If they are exercising all month and keep going as their
periods near, they report that they feel fewer and less intense PMS symptoms. Others think of exercise as energiz-

ing. A moderate exercise program doesn't drain energy; it adds energy.

Some experts recommend exercising every day. This may not be realistic for you, especially if you are just getting started. A beginning program could be only thirty to forty-five minutes a day three times a week. Spend some time scheduling your exercise, and then block out those times on your calendar. It's a safe bet that if you don't actively schedule your exercise, it won't happen.

What if you're not an athlete and you've never thought of yourself as adept at sports? With the kind of exercise we're talking about, it doesn't matter. The forms of exercise that upgrade cardiovascular fitness also seem to provide the most benefit to those with PMS. Walking briskly is all you need to do, but here's a list to get your thinking started:

—aerobics. Choose low-impact, especially if you haven't been exercising until now.

—bicycling. Get a helmet and a basket and run errands on your bike.

—swimming. This is relaxing and helpful for overall toning.

—dance. Community recreation programs offer reasonably priced classes.

—jogging. One study showed you have to jog only a minimum of 4.5 miles a week to see some improvement in PMS symptoms.

—home exercise equipment. If you have small children and it's hard to get out with them, try a stationary bicycle, a rowing machine, or a cross-country skiing machine.

—jump rope. This is cheap and easy to do at home too.

—other opportunities. Take the stairs instead of the elevator; walk to the dry cleaner's; get outside during your lunch hour.

Having an exercise partner may be helpful, especially if you're afraid you won't be able to stick with it. You can walk or jog or join an aerobics class together. If you'd rather be alone and you enjoy music, invest in an inexpensive tape player with headphones and listen as you explore new neighborhoods or hiking trails.

To avoid boredom, you can invent exercise combinations that please you and feel good to your body. You may find that walking a couple of times a week mixes well with two or three aerobics classes a week or that swimming some days and cycling others breaks the monotony of a predictable routine.

After a month or so the thirty to forty-five minutes three times a week that you started with may not seem enough. Add a day if you like. If you start with the minimum, you'll be setting yourself up for success.

YOU HAVE TO SLEEP TOO

Some women describe their feelings during their PMS days as the same as when they are extremely short on sleep, with all the jumpiness, the lassitude, the nerves that feel as if they were sticking out six feet from the body, and a rage that lurks just below the surface. Both men and women who participate in studies on sleep deprivation show surprisingly similar symptoms to women who have PMS: screaming, sobbing uncontrollably, loss of motor coordination, inaccurate perception, feelings of paranoia, and hostility.

While some women report that they have less severe PMS symptoms if they simply make time to sleep a bit more during the luteal phase of their cycles, research shows that it isn't just any old sleep that's helping. It's REM (rapid eye movement) sleep, during which we dream, that is the most restorative. In fact, it's possible to sleep for ten or eleven hours and wake up feeling bad because you never slept deeply enough to reach REM sleep. That's just the problem for some women with PMS who report more restless sleep, more awakenings, and more difficulty falling asleep again.

The small body of medical literature on sleep and PMS is inconclusive, but it's interesting to note that in one study women who had PMS reported that they dreamed more and had more dreams of a disturbing nature during their PMS times.

Unfortunately not enough investigation has yet been done in these areas to draw any broad conclusions. But these scientific musings may help you look at your own patterns and detect if getting a little more sleep during your PMS times might help you or if recording your dreams might give you some insight into what's going on in your subconscious.

TRY TO DESTRESS

Stress is what supplies the necessary edge that helps you meet a deadline or excel in an athletic event. Stress can be what makes you gobble half a box of vanilla wafers after a fight with your boyfriend, or it can be the cause of the excruciating headache you feel winding its way up from your shoulders to the back of your skull.

Positive or negative stress will have the same effect on your body. According to Debbie Takade, a California psychotherapist, "You can get fired or promoted; from the neck down, your body doesn't know the difference." That's because stress, as defined, is a stimulus that disturbs or interferes with normal physiological equilibrium. Stress triggers the production of a hormone, norepinephrine, and produces other physical effects like a stepped-up heart rate, an increase in blood pressure, sweating or icy hands, shallow breathing, an increase in gastric acid, and muscle contractions. For some women, stress also triggers more severe PMS symptoms. Many people now see that simply being alive produces stress and that you may feel the effects of it more acutely during your PMS time.

The first step toward managing the stress in your life so it doesn't manage *you* is to identify the sources of stress. Make a list, and be specific. The more you can break a problem down into particulars, the more effectively you will be able to deal with it. For example, don't just list your job as being stressful; note the lazy coworker, the long commute, the desk chair that makes your lower back ache at the end of the day.

Once you have a list, you'll be able to see how much stress in your life comes from outside yourself (traffic jams) and how much is self-imposed (trying to be all things to all people, never saying no to requests).

For those stresses you see as self-imposed, you might try:

—prioritizing tasks. Let what *can* wait, wait. You may
  feel less pressured if you don't make yourself
  accomplish everything in one day.

—setting limits. Be reasonable about what to expect from yourself, particularly during your PMS times. Try to take some time to think before you commit to doing something. If you realize that you will be able to do the things you choose to do so much better if you say no to one more commitment, it may make saying no possible.

—delegating. Do you really have to do *everything* on your list yourself? You show husband, children, and friends how much you value them and trust them if you ask them to help you out.

If most of your stress comes from outside yourself, your best solution is to get away, however briefly, from the source of the stress. You're not crazy about your new office-mate? You find your supervisor especially difficult to work with? Get out for a walk at lunchtime every day. Taking a break that removes you from the scene of the stress helps lower the overall level of stress you'll feel. If you can do it more than once a day, say, at two fifteen-minute coffee breaks *and* during lunch, so much the better.

At home create at least one little clutter-free corner for yourself. If it's a room with a door on it, terrific. Let your children know when you need a half hour of time off. If your children are too young to play independently during your breather, trade some baby-sitting time with a friend. Or arrange for your husband to give you some time alone after he comes home from work. Try a relaxation tape to replace "kid noise" with peaceful sounds. You can choose the kind that has guided meditations or simple recordings of soothing sounds from nature.

One important key to destressing your life is to incorporate relaxation techniques or breathers all through your day. What if you save up for one big exercise session at the end of the day and find out you have to stay late at the office (or at school) or you have to run your daughter to the mall for science project supplies? There goes your workout time. What if you generally are just too busy to add one more item to your schedule even if it is called "relaxing"? Debbie Takade suggests you contact a stress clinic or a reputable biofeedback specialist to help you construct small but important ways to destress all day long. Simply becoming aware of and then changing habits like gritting your teeth, squinting, chewing gum, or sitting a certain way at your computer can make a big difference.

What you eat can also make a difference in your stress level. Lowering stress goes hand in hand with lowering your consumption of sugar, salt, and caffeine, particularly during your PMS time. Make your "comfort foods" things like whole grain breads and high-fiber fruits and vegetables. With a small dietary adjustment you may see a change in how you handle the stresses you have been unable to control.

ABOUT CHANGE

If you have ever tried to change your eating or exercise habits, whether it was to lose a few pounds or just to live in a more healthy manner, you may have found that it wasn't easy. While the prospect of gaining control of your PMS may motivate you more than before, be aware that making changes will probably not be easy.

Many women find that it takes six months to a year to incorporate fully all the life-style changes they want to make. And most find that the path to change is an uneven one, running smoothly toward goals one month and bumping along with lots of ups and downs the next.

A few things you can do to set yourself up for success in your change making:

—Concentrate on making one change at a time. For example, if improving your diet seems to be the first thing you should do, focus on that for a month or two. When you begin to feel at home with dietary changes, try bringing in a reasonable walking program.

—Keep a life-style journal during this time. It doesn't have to be exhaustive; just note down what you ate, how you felt, and whether you exercised each day. Make it a continuation of the chart-keeping you began in order to see if you had PMS. After a couple of months, looking back at your journal will let you see the progress you've made and will help you evaluate which changes are working best for you.

—Give yourself credit for trying. The fact that you have taken responsibility for your health and are attempting to control your PMS is terrific in itself. Your effort will pay off. And while you're waiting for the payoff, keep yourself going by giving yourself credit for trying.

—Set realistic goals. It isn't realistic to think you'll turn your life-style upside down in a single month and that you'll keep all your resolutions without ever slipping. Lasting change happens slowly, over time. The times you don't stick to the regimen you've set for yourself can be the strongest learning times.

—Plan and begin making changes during your symptom-free days. You'll be much more likely to stick to your plan when you feel "up" and capable. And the habits you develop during the first two weeks of your cycle will eventually pull you through the difficult last two weeks.

FIVE

HORMONE THERAPY AND OTHER DRUG TREATMENTS

Although no one has found a single cause for PMS, many of the symptoms have been clearly defined. The alleviation of those symptoms is the focus of scores of medical treatments available today. As you work with the health care provider you have chosen, you may be considering one or more medical approaches to your PMS. The information here will help you understand the pros and cons of many of these. You can use this information to answer some of your questions, then to formulate additional questions for your doctor, and finally, to help you decide which treatment is right for you.

This listing of some of the most common prescription medications for PMS is grouped by the system or organ on which the medication has the greatest effect. You'll find them under these headings: hormones, diuretics, prostaglandins, psychoactive agents, antibiotics, and antifungal treatments. Surgical solutions are also discussed here.

HORMONES

Of the more than fifty suggested treatments for PMS, none has received more attention in the last couple of years than those centering on the use of hormones. And of those, progesterone has been the undisputed favorite.

Here is each of the hormone therapies in use, which of them works and for whom, and the side effects of each.

Progesterone. This hormone, which is produced by the corpus luteum during the luteal phase of the menstrual cycle, was first used to treat PMS in 1938 after a physician tried it on one of his patients. He theorized that PMS symptoms were created by a deficiency of progesterone, and his patient's symptoms improved when he gave her intramuscular injections of progesterone. He then tried the same treatment on seven women, and five of them reported their symptoms improved.

There was comment at the time that such a small, unscientific trial was hardly enough evidence on which to build a practice of prescribing progesterone for PMS, but history has proved otherwise. In 1953 Britain's Dr. Katharina Dalton began treating PMS symptoms with progesterone, and she has since treated thousands of women. Anecdotes of her success are everywhere, but as of this writing, her claims have been questioned by some in the medical community because she has never reported the results of a scientific study from her research and clinical practice.

Those who disagree with Dr. Dalton base their position on conflicting evidence about the effectiveness of progesterone and on the fact that in more than 90 percent of scientific trials done by others, progesterone was shown to be ineffective. Only one study, published in 1985, was able to show progesterone to have some beneficial effect on the twenty-three women in the study, and then primarily in the first month of treatment. Nevertheless, by the mid-1980s progesterone was the most widely recommended treatment for PMS in the United States.

Then, in July 1990, in what an editorial in the *Journal of the American Medical Association (JAMA)* called "the most convincing manner to date," progesterone was shown to be no more effective than a placebo (an inactive substance used to prove the effect of an active medication). The editorial referred to a *JAMA* report of a "carefully designed" study at the University of Pennsylvania, using dosages of progesterone recommended by Dr. Dalton and her colleagues. The sample (168 women) was larger than in any of the studies previously reported. And for the first time it pointed convincingly to the lack of effectiveness of progesterone on PMS symptoms. The investigators reported that "premenstrual symptoms were not significantly improved by progesterone compared with placebo in any measure used in the study, including daily symptom reports maintained throughout treatment, clinician evaluation of improvement and patient global reports of symptom severity, relief and disruption of daily activity. No symptom cluster or individual symptom differed significantly between progesterone and placebo treatment."

Supporters of Dr. Dalton's progesterone therapy responded that the dosages in the study were not the same as Dalton's, although the studies' investigators claim they were.

Before achieving these results, investigators on this study regularly prescribed progesterone in suppository form and stated that if they had a bias, it was that the progesterone would prove effective. They are now studying progesterone in oral form, in a trial that is scheduled to continue into 1993.

Studies notwithstanding, PMS clinics around the country that routinely prescribe progesterone report good results. Many investigators try to explain progesterone's anecdotal success by citing the education, counseling, and support that usually go along with care at a PMS clinic. They explain that it's hard to assess the effect of the progesterone separately from the effect of the support. It could be that the support helps PMS symptoms more than the hormone.

If you think you'd like to try progesterone, here are some things for you to consider:

—Cost may be an issue, depending on the form you use and the pharmaceutical company your physician buys from. Prices for a year's worth of four-hundred-milligram (mg) suppositories (taken daily for fourteen days a month) can range from two hundred to two thousand dollars a year depending on the manufacturer. Oral tablets or capsules may run from three hundred to four hundred dollars a year.

—If you use progesterone, be sure you are getting the natural, as opposed to the synthetic, form. Natural progesterone comes in suppositories and in an oral form that is micronized, to keep it from being inactivated by the liver. Anecdotal evidence shows that synthetic progesterone, or progestin, is less effective than natural, and trials clearly show the synthetic has far more serious side effects. Oral progestin has been shown to cause such blood-clotting disorders as thrombophlebitis and blood clots in the heart and brain. It may also cause birth defects, bleeding, spotting, edema (bloating), amenorrhea (cessation of menstrual periods), depression, nausea, and sleep problems. In contrast, the primary reported side effect of natural progesterone has been drowsiness.

—In some women natural progesterone has been shown to *induce* PMS symptoms that were not present before.

—The basis for using progesterone has never been proved—namely, that women who have PMS have a deficiency of the hormone or an excess of estrogen, which causes an imbalance between that and progesterone.

*Oral Contraceptives. Oral contraceptives, or birth control pills, contain a combination of various synthetic estrogens and progestins that keep you from getting pregnant by inhibiting the surge of hormones that would normally cause ovulation.

Research on whether the pill is effective for PMS symptoms is equivocal. Several large-scale surveys show that depression and irritability may be reduced with oral contraceptive use. Other studies show that some women stopped taking the pill because they developed those symptoms while on it. Several studies did show that there were less severe symptoms for women who took *combination* pills, in which some amount of each hormone was taken in combination with the other all month, compared with those who took *sequential* pills, in which one hormone followed the other.

A major consideration for women who take birth control pills is the pill's side effects, especially for women who smoke. Thromboembolism, stroke, and heart attack are more common in women who take the pill. It can also cause depression, fluid retention, gastrointestinal distress, breast changes, and vaginal bleeding.

Antiestrogen. An antiestrogen is an oral drug that competes for estrogen binding sites in specific organs such as the breast. One antiestrogen, called tamoxifen (sold as Nolvadex), which is usually used to treat breast cancer in postmenopausal women, has been studied for use in women whose major PMS symptoms are breast-related. One study showed that it certainly relieved breast tenderness, or mastalgia, far better than the placebo. But drawbacks of this drug are that it has not been studied for use on any other PMS symptoms, and it has some nasty side effects, including hot flushes, nausea, vomiting, menstrual irregularities, and vaginal bleeding. It also may cause fetal harm if you become pregnant while using it.

Danazol. This is a synthetic androgen, or male hormone, that affects the communication between the hypothalamus, pituitary, and ovaries in order to suppress ovulation. Danazol (sold as Danocrine) is often used to treat endometriosis. It was first studied as a treatment for PMS in 1979 on the premise that if you didn't have the various hormones' cycles that produced your menstrual period, you wouldn't have PMS. Several studies have followed, with two showing that after three months of taking 200 mg of danazol a day, several PMS symptoms (depression, aggression, lethargy, anxiety, tearfulness, irritability, and breast pain) were improved.

However, many studies were plagued by dropouts because danazol is not well tolerated by the majority of women, and in an overview of all the studies, the only symptom fairly reliably relieved was breast pain. Side effects for danazol are what you might expect from taking male hormones: increased hairiness on the face and chest, decreased breast size, vaginitis, nausea, and weight gain. In addition, danazol should not be taken by women contemplating pregnancy, already pregnant, or nursing, or by women who have liver, kidney, or heart problems.

Testosterone. This is the major male hormone, which accounts for sperm production, among other things. In women testosterone is produced in small amounts in the ovaries and adrenal glands, and it modulates libido.

Testosterone was first used to treat PMS in 1940 and has been studied off and on since then, as recently as 1984, but never rigorously. It has been used on the premise that PMS symptoms are caused by excess estrogens and that more testosterone would neutralize them. Indeed, each time it has been tested, it has worked pretty well, relieving symptoms of tension, irritability, anxiety, depression, and bloating. However, some women who participated in studies found their periods delayed, and others found that their periods stopped altogether. For most women, these side effects stopped when they stopped taking the hormone. But for some, who took a synthetic form of testosterone called anabolic steroids, side effects such as increased facial hair, deep voices, and male-looking physiques were permanent.

Testosterone presents serious risks to the fetus if you should become pregnant while taking it.

GnRH Agonist. These chemicals work against gonadotropin-releasing hormone (GnRH), which normally plays a big part in stimulating the menstrual cycle. The result is that within two to four weeks of treatment the amount of estrogen you produce is reduced to postmenopausal levels and your menstrual cycle stops.

One GnRH agonist in use is leuprolide acetate (sold as Lupron), which is given by injection.

GnRH agonists present two serious problems:

—While the loss of the menstrual cycle during treatment is reversible, no one knows what the long-term effects of that temporary loss are.

—Reducing estrogens to postmenopausal levels could lead to an increased risk of osteoporosis.

Thyroid Hormone. Some in the medical community have postulated that women with PMS may really be suffering from an underlying thyroid problem. Indeed, thyroid disorder is one of the common misdiagnoses for PMS. One 1986 study showed that of fifty-four women with PMS, thirty-five (69 percent), when tested, were found to have a low-level thyroid dysfunction. Of thirty-four who were treated, all experienced complete relief of symptoms when given levothyroxine sodium, a synthetic form of thyroid hormone (sold as Synthroid).

It might be a good idea to have your thyroid function assessed by a simple blood test at your doctor's office.

Prolactin-Related Treatment. This has been studied and used for the last six or eight years under the premise that PMS symptoms, particularly breast symptoms, are the result of high concentrations of prolactin, the hormone that helps produce breast milk. The drug used is bromocriptine (sold as Parlodel), which is most often prescribed to curtail the flow of breast milk in mothers who choose not to nurse their babies. While bromocriptine did get rid of breast tenderness and swelling, every study using it reported adverse side effects, ranging from mild (nausea, headache, dizziness, and fatigue) to extremely serious (dramatic changes in blood pressure, seizures, strokes, heart attacks, blood clots, and psychosis).

DIURETICS

Some medical references call diuretics the most over-prescribed medication for PMS. Research shows that despite the puffy, bloated feeling a woman may have, unless she can tell objectively—that is, by the scale—that she regularly gains several pounds premenstrually and loses them during her period, the bloated feeling is due most likely to redistribution of body fluids, not to additional body fluids. Some in the medical community who prescribe diuretics for PMS believe that besides avoiding premenstrual weight gain, diuretics help relieve premenstrual headaches and irritability, but there have been no studies that show diuretics to have that effect.

Spironolactone. If actual, regular weight gain is occurring, the diuretic of choice is spironolactone, primarily because it does not deplete the body of potassium as other diuretics may. Its side effects include: gastrointestinal disturbance, central nervous system depression, and irregular periods. It has been shown to cause tumors in rats, and it should not be used during pregnancy.

Ammonium Chloride. This is not used alone but as an ingredient in diuretic products. This drug does seem to limit bloating, but it has not been studied rigorously, so it's not clear whether its long-term use is safe or advisable. It apparently has no effect on menstrually related migraine or painful breasts and must be used for two or three months for its effect to be evident.

Thiazide. In some studies this drug had a good effect on swelling, but it can also affect the electrolyte balance in your body because it depletes potassium. Some experts think that if you're going to take a diuretic, it shouldn't be one that depletes potassium.

Metolazone, Chlorthalidone, Triamterene. All these have been studied at least to a small degree for use in PMS. All carry the same precautions as thiazide diuretics, including the fact that they have no effect unless you actually gain weight premenstrually. They do nothing to relieve a bloated feeling.

PROSTAGLANDIN-RELATED TREATMENT

As you may recall from Chapter 2, prostaglandins are chemicals produced by the endometrium when the progesterone level falls at the end of the luteal phase and the beginning of the menstrual period. It appears that the production of prostaglandins is the cause of the pain and nausea that accompany menstruation for some women. More recent studies have been conducted on the premise that prostaglandins may also produce PMS symptoms.

A drug called mefenamic acid (sold as Ponstel) has been studied for its possible effect on PMS symptoms. It was effective only on the symptoms related to pain. Some health care providers question the validity of prescribing this drug because it received mixed reviews on whether it addresses the major PMS symptoms (like depression, breast tenderness, tension, irritability, and fluid retention) and because the drug has bothersome side effects (rash, diarrhea, and other gastrointestinal disturbances).

PSYCHOACTIVE AGENTS

These are drugs that affect your mood, and there are many different types. Current conventional wisdom is that if psychoactive drugs are used for PMS, their use should be for the short term only, unless the woman has a preexisting affective disorder (like clinical depression, for example, a disorder that is present all the time, not just during the luteal phase of her cycle). Some women find some of these drugs helpful in the short term as they learn to control their PMS symptoms using other methods. But for many women, being given a psychoactive drug when they seek help for PMS is the same as the physician's saying, "It's all in your head," because these drugs don't address the physical realities of PMS.

Of perhaps even greater concern are the serious side effects, including addiction, produced by some of these drugs. Many physicians would agree that psychoactive drugs should not be the treatment of first resort. Others will write out a prescription as soon as you mention the word *depression*. To help you know your options, here are some of the psychoactive drugs that may be prescribed for PMS:

Antianxiety drugs. These include alprazolam (sold as Xanax), meprobamate (sold as Miltown), and buspirone (sold as BuSpar).

Alprazolam has been used to treat PMS symptoms of anxiety, tension, and insomnia. However, because it acts as a sedative (you cannot drive or use alcohol while taking this), it is unsafe to take it during pregnancy, and its side effects include bone and joint stiffness, labored breathing, visual problems, profuse sweating, and rapidly alternating mood swings. In addition, you may develop a tolerance/dependence situation, in which more of the drug is needed to maintain the same effect. Withdrawal from the drug is difficult, requiring a slow tapering off under psychiatric supervision.

Meprobamate has been used since the 1950s to treat anxiety. But both physical and psychological dependence can occur with this drug, along with an impairment of mental and physical abilities. Meprobamate also interacts with alcohol and other central nervous system depressants, so its use must be carefully monitored. Side effects include drowsiness, weakness, nausea, headache, tachycardia (rapid heartbeat), and allergic reaction. It has been linked to an increased risk of birth defects in the first trimester.

Buspirone is a relatively new drug, also used to treat anxiety. There is some concern that long-term use may lead to motor dysfunction, but it has not been in use long enough to be certain.

Antidepressants. These include nortriptyline (sold as Pamelor) and fluoxetine (sold as Prozac).

According to some sources, Prozac, approved by the FDA in 1987, is the most prescribed antidepressant in America, even though it costs considerably more than other antidepressants. It apparently works by blocking the reabsorption of the neurotransmitter serotonin, keeping it in circulation. Used primarily to treat depression, Prozac is also prescribed to treat addictions, bulimia, and obsessive-compulsive disorder. While some call Prozac a "miracle drug," partly because its physical side effects (headache, nausea, and nervousness) are mild compared with other antidepressants, critics aren't nearly so enthusiastic. Roughly sixty lawsuits are pending against Eli Lilly & Co., the pharmaceutical company that manufactures Prozac, because of suicide attempts and homicides committed by people while taking the drug. A Harvard study found that six patients using Prozac suffered "violent suicidal preoccupation," and there have been scores of other complaints to the manufacturer against the drug. In addition, long-term effects of the drug are not known because it has been on the market for such a short time.

Some women in studies using nortriptyline (Pamelor) reported being less depressed during their PMS times, but side effects were strong enough that others dropped out of the studies. Side effects include confusional states, insomnia, palpitations, dry mouth, skin rash, nausea, breast enlargement, urinary frequency, and fatigue. Toxic overdoses have been reported, and those taking it must avoid alcohol and be extremely careful driving or operating machinery because physical and mental abilities may be impaired. The safe use of this drug during pregnancy has not been established.

Another type of antidepressant called monoamine oxidase (MAO) inhibitors (sold as Marplan and Nardil, among others) has been suggested as a treatment for premenstrual depression, most likely because they are used to treat clinical depression. No trials have been done on their use for PMS, and those who take these must follow a carefully controlled diet, limiting cheese, yogurt, smoked meats, and alcohol, among other foods and drinks. Drugs of this category can induce serious increases in blood pressure, and their safe use during pregnancy has not been established.

Antimania Drugs. These are used in the treatment of manic episodes and include drugs such as lithium (sold as Eskalith), clonidine (sold as Catapres), and verapamil (sold as Isoptin). Clonidine and verapamil are primarily used to control hypertension and cardiac arrhythmias, respectively, but they also have been known to have an effect on some PMS symptoms like anxiety and tension. None of these drugs has been extensively studied for use in PMS, so it is not known what their effects are on any but a few psychological symptoms like anxiety, aggressiveness, and irritability. All have considerable side effects, including hand tremors, diarrhea, drowsiness, muscle weakness, and birth defects (lithium); drowsiness and high blood pressure on withdrawal (clonidine); confusion, insomnia, and psychotic symptoms (verapamil).

Tranquilizers. Bellergal is a combination drug including a possibly habit-forming barbiturate, thought to work by decreasing the activity of both the parasympathetic and the sympathetic nervous systems. It is often used to treat menopausal symptoms like hot flushes, cardiovascular disorders like palpitation and tachycardia, and gastrointestinal disorders. One study showed that after three months on Bellergal, subjects saw significant improvement in PMS symptoms of fatigue, nervousness, tender breasts, irritability, lethargy, and listlessness.

However, Bellergal can change the muscle tone of the uterus, and it is not suggested for women who wish to have children. Other side effects are blurred vision, urinary retention, dry mouth, among others.

Anorectics. Testing on an obesity drug called fenfluramine (sold as Pondimin) has shown that it reduces PMS depression in some women by affecting serotonin, a major transmitter chemical in the brain. Testing is continuing at the Massachusetts Institute of Technology to discern further the role of serotonin in PMS. Pondimin may produce psychological dependence, high doses are toxic, and its use may cause diarrhea, sedation, and depression. It should not be used with blood pressure medication or alcohol.

ANTIBIOTICS

One school of thought holds that PMS symptoms are caused by a low-grade infection within the genital tract. A study has shown improvement of PMS symptoms in women given doxycycline (sold as Vibramycin, among others), which is a form of tetracycline. Problems with this are that in the study the antibiotic was given every day throughout the cycle, a regimen that many physicians would question. In addition, it's a problem if you get pregnant while you are taking it: At worst, tetracycline has been shown in animal studies to be toxic to embryos; at best, it can permanently stain the teeth of the developing fetus. Side effects include supergrowth of yeast or other fungi, sensitivity to sunlight, and some gastrointestinal distress.

ANTIFUNGAL TREATMENTS

Another school of thought lays the blame for PMS symptoms at the feet of systemic yeast infections, but once again, lack of thorough study leaves even the investigators with a question mark instead of an answer. One study, in which women were treated with nystatin (sold as Mycostatin), which is active against yeast and other fungi, showed many physical PMS symptoms improved, with the exception of depression, the major complaint of participants. Nystatin can be taken during pregnancy.

SURGERY

Almost everyone would agree that a surgical approach to PMS should be truly an effort of last resort, made only after every other treatment has been tried and only when PMS symptoms are so debilitating as to be totally intolerable.

While at times it may be tempting to think that life would be easier if you just didn't have to deal with the parts of your body that are sometimes hard to live with, keep in mind that surgery is not a magical cure for PMS. In understanding what a surgical approach can and cannot offer, you must first understand the terminology used to define different surgeries:

—partial (or subtotal) hysterectomy. This surgery is rarely performed today. In this procedure, the uterus is removed, but the ovaries, Fallopian tubes, and cervix remain. Your hormones continue to cycle, but because you have no uterus, you no longer have menstrual periods. Women who have had partial hysterectomies still need to have yearly Pap smears to ascertain the health of their cervixes.

—total hysterectomy. Contrary to how this term sounds, the uterus and cervix are removed, but the ovaries and the Fallopian tubes remain. As with a partial hysterectomy, hormonal cycling and ovulation continue, with released eggs being absorbed into the pelvic cavity.

—total hysterectomy with bilateral salpingo-oophorectomy. The uterus, cervix, Fallopian tubes (salpingo), and both ovaries (oophor) all are removed. *Bilateral* means the ovaries and tubes from both sides are removed; in some cases only those from one side are removed.

—radical hysterectomy. This is usually performed only in cases of widespread cancer. In this surgery the uterus, the Fallopian tubes, the ovaries, the upper part of the vagina, and possibly the lymph nodes in the groin are removed.

—oophorectomy or ovariectomy. Only the ovaries are removed.

Of these types of surgery, only those removing both ovaries would have an effect on PMS. As explained in Chapter 2, the cycling of hormones produced in the ovaries seems to have the greatest effect on PMS. Generally, if you don't have the hormones and their cycles, you don't have PMS.

However, there are many important considerations linked to having your ovaries removed. One is that anecdotal evidence (but no formal studies) shows that a few women *still* have PMS symptoms even after removal of their ovaries. Despite the fact that symptoms without hormones flies in the face of reason, the anecdotal evidence exists.

Also, removal of your ovaries instantly produces what is called surgical menopause. If you have not gone through menopause already, the sudden withdrawal of estrogen produced by your ovaries will bring on menopausal symptoms you may not have bargained for, like hot flushes and vaginal dryness. And there is evidence that surgical menopause may cause even greater bone loss (leading to osteoporosis) than that which occurs after natural menopause.

A third consideration is that hysterectomy removes the uterus and ovaries and is major abdominal surgery. If only the uterus is removed, it can be taken out through the vagina, a procedure that is easier on the patient, but not all surgeons are adept at this. Removal of more than the uterus generally means an abdominal incision.

Other side effects of hysterectomy, particularly when the ovaries are also removed, are:

—an increased risk of heart disease.

—fatigue, insomnia, urinary tract problems, joint pain, headaches, and dizziness.

—lack of sexual interest and desire after surgery. Ovaries secrete up to half of a woman's supply of androgens, or male hormones (the rest comes from the adrenal glands), which are responsible for her sex drive.

—depression, related to estrogen deprivation.

In addition, about 10 percent of women undergoing hysterectomy will lose enough blood to require a transfusion, and complication (fever and bleeding) rates after hysterectomy range up to 50 percent in some areas.

Estrogen replacement therapy may take care of many of the aftereffects of hysterectomy, but not all women can tolerate it. And there is concern that estrogen therapy may increase the risk of breast cancer.

If you have only your uterus, not your ovaries, removed, you will likely still have the same PMS symptoms you had before surgery, but now you won't have a predictable PMS cycle because you no longer have periods. Many women who have had this kind of surgery claim that their PMS symptoms have worsened or that the surgery has triggered PMS symptoms they never had before. No studies have been done on this, and some physicians explain these complaints by pointing to the lack of predictability, which they say can make the same symptoms *seem* worse.

Tubal ligation, a means of permanent contraception selected by millions of American women each year, also does nothing to stop PMS symptoms. This surgery involves cauterizing (burning), clipping, or tying off the Fallopian tubes so that a mature egg cannot come into contact with sperm and be fertilized.

In anecdotal evidence similar to that connected with hysterectomies, some women believe that their PMS started or got worse after a tubal ligation.

FOOD SUPPLEMENTS AND ALTERNATIVE TREATMENTS

In its attempts to control PMS symptoms, conventional medicine has come up with approaches that in hindsight can seem pretty extreme, from "tuning" the ovaries with X-ray treatments in the 1930s to removing them altogether in the 1990s.

If the medical approaches in the previous chapter don't appeal to you, or if you've tried some of them to no avail, you may be interested in the following alternative approaches.

Some alternative approaches have grown out of traditional concoctions like Lydia Pinkham's Vegetable Compound. If you were a woman with PMS living in the late nineteenth century, you might have swallowed a lot of Miss Pinkham's compound—a then popular remedy for PMS.

Today, while some people may assume Lydia Pinkham's mixture was useless because it wasn't "scientific," the mainstream medical world has begun to recognize that many herbal or folk remedies like hers did help some PMS symptoms. For example, Lydia may not have known that the black cohosh she used in her compound contained estrogen, but experience showed her that black cohosh along with the other herbs she added relieved PMS symptoms for many women.

The same kind of experiential knowledge about vitamins has been around a long time too. In many cases the effect produced by eating certain foods was known long before the responsible vitamin was named. And the *effect* is why, before you look at vitamins and herbs as treatments for PMS, it's important to see them as powerful substances. Just because you don't need a prescription for any of these, it doesn't mean they can't have a strong impact, maybe even a negative one if you use too much.

As with medications in the previous chapter, possible toxicity and side effects are included in the discussions of substances listed here. The Resource List (in the back of this book) includes the names of some reference books you might like to consult for more information, and you might want to talk to a qualified herbalist or nutritional consultant too. How to find either of those is also in the Resource List.

VITAMINS

In Chapter 4 you read about certain foods containing nutrients that help many women with PMS symptoms. If you would like to focus on a particular PMS symptom, like acne, for example, you could eat more of the foods that contain the nutrients (vitamin A, in this case) that can help the symptom, and you can add vitamin supplements to your diet.

Certain vitamins have been more helpful for PMS symptoms than others. They are:

Vitamin A. This fat-soluble vitamin is particularly good for the skin, for helping your eyes see in the dark, and for growth. It is stored in the liver and metabolized slowly. The recommended daily allowance (RDA) is four thousand international units (IU) in nonpregnant, nonlactating women. Chronic toxicity can occur at doses of fifty thousand units per day for longer than eighteen months, or five hundred thousand units daily for two months. Toxicity symptoms include hair loss, nausea, vomiting, diarrhea, scaly skin, blurred vision, rashes, bone pain, irregular menstrual periods, fatigue, headaches, and liver enlargement.

Vitamin A was first used for PMS in the late 1940s and then tested in the 1950s and 1960s. In two studies, women took two hundred thousand to three hundred thousand units of the vitamin daily from day 15 of their cycles until their periods began. After three to four months 80 to 100 percent of the women said that their symptoms of bloating, breast tenderness, and nervous tension were greatly improved.

While it's good news that vitamin A seemed to have such a positive effect, the dosages in the studies were very high. A more recent suggested therapeutic level of vitamin A is 15,000 IU a day. You might discuss this with a physician, or consider adding vitamin A-rich foods to your diet along with a more reasonable supplement.

Best natural sources: Vitamin A is found in natural fish liver oil and plant sources (from which it is not toxic in large doses). Some foods that are good sources of vitamin A are salmon, carrots, butternut squash, dandelion greens, Hubbard squash, sweet potatoes, turnip greens, kale, bok choy, broccoli, sweet red peppers, apricots, romaine lettuce, peaches, asparagus, butter lettuce.

B Vitamins. These are water-soluble and are not stored for long periods in the body, so they must be replenished regularly. Emotional stress can speed the loss of vitamins B_1, $_2$, and $_3$, resulting in irritability and fatigue. In all, there are eleven B vitamins, but four of them (B_1, B_2, B_3, and B_6) seem to have the greatest effect on PMS symptoms. However, since all eleven need one another in order for any of them to work, if you decide you need one or two as supplements, you must take the rest too.

Pyridoxine, vitamin B_6. Many women report improvement in PMS symptoms like food cravings, fluid retention, irritability, breast tenderness, fatigue, and mood swings when they take large doses of B_6 premenstrually. Vitamin B_6 may be necessary for neurotransmitters like serotonin to function properly, and it plays a part in the metabolism of protein and carbohydrates. However, results of some studies on B_6 are inconclusive and contradictory, showing that it helps moderate symptoms in some women but not in others. In addition, several studies showed that even though B_6 is a water-soluble vitamin that passes from the body relatively quickly, large doses can be toxic, producing neurological disorders, night restlessness, and too-vivid dream recall. Doses over 500 mg daily are not recommended; RDA for B_6 is 1.8 to 2.2 mg daily, with higher doses during pregnancy and lactation. Therapeutic doses for PMS are 200 to 500 mg daily, taken with meals and in combination with a B complex vitamin.

Best natural sources: brewer's yeast, wheat bran, wheat germ, liver, cantaloupe, cabbage, blackstrap molasses, milk, eggs.

Thiamine, vitamin B_1. This vitamin is known as the morale vitamin because of its beneficial effects on the nervous system and mental attitude. The RDA is 1.0 to 1.5 mg. High-potency doses for PMS range from 50 to 500 mg. It is not known to be toxic.

Best natural sources: dried yeast, rice husk, whole wheat, oatmeal, peanuts, pork, most vegetables, bran, milk.

Riboflavin, vitamin B_2: In the United States the most common vitamin deficiency is in riboflavin, which, like other B vitamins, is especially important if you are under stress. The RDA is 1.2 to 1.7 mg, with a higher-potency dose for PMS ranging from 100 to 300 mg. Though B_2 has no known toxic effects, possible symptoms of overuse are itching, numbness, and a burning or prickling sensation of the skin.

Best natural sources: milk, liver, kidney, yeast, cheese, leafy green vegetables, fish, eggs.

Niacin, vitamin B_3. Vitamin B_3 is necessary for healthy nervous system and brain function and for the synthesis of sex hormones, among other things. The RDA is 13 to 19 mg; 50 to 100 mg daily for PMS. B_3 is not known to be toxic, but skin flushing along with a burning or itching sensation may occur at daily doses over 100 mg.

Best natural sources: liver, lean meat, whole wheat products, brewer's yeast, kidney, wheat germ, fish, eggs.

*Vitamin E. Unlike other fat-soluble vitamins, E is stored in the body for a short time, so it must be replenished daily by foods or supplements. Vitamin E helps alleviate fatigue, aids in healing, supplies oxygen to the body for greater endurance, and acts as a mild diuretic. Some women feel it helps premenstrual breast tenderness, and studies have shown it effective against headache, fatigue, insomnia, depression, and food cravings. The RDA for vitamin E is 30 IU; 300 to 600 IU daily for PMS. Vitamin E doesn't appear to be toxic at these doses, but some toxicity has occurred in doses over 8,000 IU per day.

Best natural sources: wheat germ, soybean, vegetable oil, broccoli, brussels sprouts, leafy green vegetables, spinach, enriched flour, whole wheat, whole grain cereal, eggs.

Vitamin C. This water-soluble vitamin is used up more rapidly when you are under stress, so you may want to increase your intake premenstrually. The RDA for vitamin C is 45 mg; PMS dosage is 500 mg to 3 g. If you take a high dose of vitamin C daily, you run a risk of kidney stone formation, so be sure you drink a lot of water to keep your system cleansed, and add a magnesium supplement to help guard against kidney stones.

Best natural sources: citrus fruits, berries, leafy green vegetables, tomatoes, cauliflower, potatoes, sweet potatoes.

OTHER SUPPLEMENTS

Minerals, dietary fiber, amino acids, and essential fatty acids all have a place in easing certain PMS symptoms. In addition, several pharmaceutical companies now produce over-the-counter preparations directed at PMS symptoms. As with all approaches for PMS, no single one of these offers relief from all symptoms, but many can help with individual symptoms. Use this list to find which of these supplements may help you.

Magnesium. This mineral is essential for effective nerve and muscle functioning. It is also known as the anti-stress mineral because it helps fight depression. Several researchers advocate the use of magnesium for PMS on the premise that some women who had PMS were found to be deficient premenstrually in plasma magnesium concentrations. However, magnesium supplements have not been studied alone, so their effectiveness remains to be determined. It is often a part of multivitamins, particularly those specified for PMS. The RDA for magnesium is 300 to 450 mg; slightly more for PMS.

Best natural sources: figs, lemons, grapefruit, yellow corn, almonds, nuts, seeds, dark green vegetables, apples.

Dietary fiber. On the basis of the theory that PMS symptoms result from excess estrogen, some health care providers recommend increasing dietary fiber consumption to 20 to 40 grams a day to increase fecal excretion, thereby increasing estrogen excretion too. During the 1930s laxatives were sometimes prescribed for PMS for the same reason. However, no studies have been done to show that more dietary fiber results in lower plasma estrogen concentrations, and no studies have shown that lower estrogen levels mean no PMS symptoms. On the other hand, it wouldn't hurt to increase the fiber in your diet. The National Cancer Institute of the National Institutes of Health advocates consuming twenty to thirty grams of fiber a day, and if you find more dietary fiber helps your PMS, so much the better.

Best natural sources: whole grains and whole grain products, fresh fruits and vegetables. Foods to avoid are highly processed or refined grains and their products.

Amino Acids. L-tryptophan is an amino acid essential for the synthesis of the neurotransmitter serotonin. Decreased serotonin can account for depression and other psychological symptoms of PMS, and more than one researcher has theorized that the lack of serotonin may play an underlying role in causing PMS. But the theory that some kind of disruption in the process of normal serotonin secretion causes PMS, along with the idea that oral tryptophan supplements can affect the synthesis of a neurotransmitter, has yet to be proved.

For a while in the late 1980s L-tryptophan supplements were being prescribed for PMS symptoms, and anecdotal information showed it relieved psychological symptoms for some women. However, by late 1989 and early 1990 many women taking L-tryptophan had become ill with what turned out to be a rare and sometimes fatal blood disorder. By mid-1990 twenty-one deaths, along with about fifteen hundred cases of the blood disorder, called eosinophilia myalgia, had been reported. Consequently, the Food and Drug Administration recalled all brands of the amino acid as it researched the cause of the disorder. As of mid-1991 the recall was still in effect while studies on the amino acid progressed.

Essential Fatty Acids. Evening primrose oil, culled from the flower, contains the essential fatty acid linoleic acid, which apparently increases the body's output of a certain kind of prostaglandin. Theories hold that the boost in prostaglandins lowers prolactin levels, alleviating PMS symptoms for some women. Studies haven't proved this theory, but some women find relief by taking evening primrose oil in capsule form.

OVER-THE-COUNTER PREPARATIONS

You may have noticed that since the early 1980s, when PMS "came out" as a legitimate problem, the shelf at your local pharmacy that used to hold only Midol, Pamprin, and aspirin now holds much more. Generally, over-the-counter PMS preparations fall into three categories:

—*Combination drugs.* These usually contain an analgesic, a diuretic, and an antihistamine. Use of the antihistamine is partially based on a 1950s theory that some PMS symptoms occur because of an allergy to one's own hormones. As a result, the body produces histamines, which in turn cause some PMS symptoms, like irritability. Many investigators believe this theory is not supported by current research. Pharmaceutical companies justify their use of antihistamines by pointing to studies done within their laboratories that show that the antihistamine pyrilamine maleate helped reduce irritability and water retention. The FDA has lent "reserved" support to their findings, requiring that antihistamines be used for PMS only in combination with at least one other drug shown more conclusively to relieve PMS symptoms.

—*Diuretics.* These work only on the symptom of bloatedness, but some women who experience actual weight gain premenstrually also report improvement in their moods when their water retention is eliminated.

—*Nutritional supplements.* These include many of the vitamins and offer dietary supplements listed earlier in this chapter.

While the over-the-counter preparations listed here have been approved by the Food and Drug Administration, it's important to know that the FDA does not require manufacturers to distinguish clearly between the terms *premenstrual* and *menstrual* in describing products. Consequently, combination drugs advertised as being for PMS symptoms contain an analgesic—a pain reliever—when by definition, pain is not a PMS symptom.

If you want to try an over-the-counter product, be sure to read the label so that you know what you are (and aren't) getting.

Here is a table of the most common PMS preparations:

Over-the-Counter PMS Preparations

Name	Manufacturer	Active Ingredient and Its Action
COMBINATION DRUGS		
Lurline PMS	Fielding	acetaminophen (analgesic) pamabrom (diuretic) pyridoxine (vitamin B_6)
Maximum Strength Midol PMS	Glenbrook	acetaminophen (analgesic) pamabrom (diuretic) pyrilamine maleate (antihistamine)
Pamprin Multi-Symptom Extra-Strength Pain Relief Formula Tablets	Chattem	Same as above
Premsyn PMS	Chattem	Same as above
Pursettes PMS Tablets	Jeffrey Martin	Same as above
DIURETICS		
Aqua-Ban	Thompson	ammonium chloride (325 mg diuretic) caffeine (100 mg diuretic, stimulant)
Aqua-Ban Maximum Strength	Thompson	ammonium chloride (650 mg, diuretic) caffeine (200 mg. diuretic, stimulant)
Ordinil Water Pill	Fox Pharmacal	pamabrom (diuretic)

Name	Manufacturer	Active Ingredient and Its Action
NUTRITIONAL SUPPLEMENTS		
Efamol PMS	Nature's Way Products	vitamin B_6 vitamin E vitamin C calcium magnesium zinc natural oil base
Neurovites	Flanders	vitamin A vitamin E vitamin D vitamins B_1, B_2, B_3, B_6, B_{12}, folic acid biotin pantothenic acid choline inositol PABA citrus bioflavonoid vitamin C rutin calcium magnesium iodine iron zinc copper manganese potassium selenium chromium pancreatin betaine
Optivite	Optimox, Inc.	vitamin A vitamin E vitamin D_3 folic acid

Name	Manufacturer	Active Ingredient and Its Action
		vitamin B$_1$
		vitamin B$_2$
		niacinamide
		vitamin B$_6$
		vitamin B$_{12}$
		pantothenic acid (B$_5$)
		choline bitartrate
		vitamin C
		magnesium
		iodine
		iron
		copper
		zinc
		manganese
		potassium
		selenium
		chromium
PMS Balance: Premenstrual Nutrition Supplement	Rexall Nutritional Products	vitamin B$_6$ vitamin E magnesium
ProCycle	Madison Pharmacy Associates	vitamin A
		vitamin E
		vitamin D$_3$
		folic acid
		vitamin B$_1$
		vitamin B$_2$
		vitamin B$_6$
		vitamin B$_{12}$
		biotin
		niacinamide
		pantothenic acid
		choline bitartrate
		inositol
		para-aminobenzoic acid
		vitamin C
		bioflavonoids

Name	Manufacturer	Active Ingredient and Its Action
		rutin
		calcium
		magnesium
		iodine
		iron
		copper
		zinc
		manganese
		potassium
		selenium
		chromium
Windmill Pre-Menstrual Supplement	Windmill Vitamin Company	evening primrose oil
		vitamin B_6
		magnesium
		calcium
		potassium
		folic acid
		herbal complex base

HERBS

For thousands of years herbs have been used for their medicinal properties. The idea behind herbal medicine is to stimulate the body's own defenses rather than treat symptoms only.

Please keep in mind that we are not recommending specific herbal remedies for PMS symptoms. It is difficult to find a qualified herbalist or naturopathic physician (ND), and it is certainly unwise to attempt self-treatment. Nonetheless, some women report that herbal remedies have relieved their symptoms, so we are including an overview of herbal medicine for information only.

Herbs are taken in many ways, but the most typical for those described here are infusions, decoctions, or tinctures.

Infusions. These are extracts made from herbs with medicinal qualities in their flowers, stems, and leaves. Infusions differ from teas in that they are steeped longer to become considerably stronger. Traditionally an infusion calls for one-half to one ounce of a dried herb (or double the amount for fresh) steeped in a pint of boiling water for up to twenty minutes.

Decoctions. These are similar to infusions, but they are made from roots and barks that must be simmered for ten to twenty minutes in order to extract the necessary chemicals.

Tinctures. These are highly concentrated extracts of herbs made with alcohol rather than water. You can learn to make your own, but it may be easier to buy tinctures from a good health food store or from one of the sources listed in the Resource List (in the back of the book).

Herbs can be powerful substances. Be sure to:

—use only recommended amounts of the herb for recommended periods of time. As with other drugs, it is *not* true that if a little is good, more will be better.

—start with low-strength preparations if you are sensitive to other drugs.

—be extra cautious if you have a chronic disease or if you take other medications. Drugs can interact with healing herbs.

—pay attention to symptoms of toxicity. If you develop stomach upset, nausea, diarrhea, or headache within an hour of taking a healing herb, do not take another dose. If symptoms do not subside, call your herbalist, physician, or local poison control center.

—use herbs only in consultation with your physician. Many herbs can interact with drugs or have an effect you may not be aware of on another part of your body.

Herbs typically used for PMS address four symptoms or groups of symptoms: bloating, depression, mental acuity, and anxiety.

Bloating. Many of the healing herbs, including buchu, celery seed, uva-ursi, dandelion, juniper, nettle, parsley, and sarsaparilla, act as diuretics. As with the diuretics discussed in the previous chapter, these may also deplete your body of potassium if taken over a long period of time. If you use any of these herbs, increase your intake of potassium by eating more bananas, tomatoes, and leafy green vegetables.

One of the most effective herbal diuretics is buchu, also called the South African water pill. Natives of Namibia and South Africa used the leaves of this shrub long before contact with European settlers. Today buchu is an ingredient in two over-the-counter diuretics.

For relief of PMS bloating, use an infusion or tincture. For an infusion, steep one to two teaspoons of dried, crumbled leaves per cup of boiling water for ten to twenty minutes. Drink three cups a day. In a tincture take one-half to one teaspoon up to three times a day. If buchu causes stomach upset or diarrhea, use less or stop using it.

Depression. The herb that stands out as most effective against depression is St.-John's-wort, although motherwort and celery seed have also been used. Studies have shown that St.-John's-wort contains a substance called hypericin that appears to interfere with the activity of the body chemical monoamine oxidase (MAO), making it an MAO inhibitor. MAO inhibitors are an important class of antidepressants and form the basis of several pharmaceutical products. St.-John's-wort is not known to work instantly; the effect develops over two or three months.

For relief from PMS-related depression, make an infusion of from one to two teaspoons of dried herb per cup of boiling water. Steep for ten to fifteen minutes, and drink up to three cups a day. In a tincture use one-fourth to one teaspoon up to three times a day.

While St.-John's-wort is not as powerful as its pharmaceutical counterparts, it's a good idea to follow similar precautions when taking it. If you develop headache, stiff neck, or nausea, stop taking it and consult your physician. While you are taking St.-John's-wort, do not take amphetamines, narcotics, the amino acids tryptophan and tyrosine, diet pills, asthma inhalants, nasal decongestants, or cold or hay fever medication. In addition, don't eat preserved meats and pickled or smoked items; don't drink wine, beer, or coffee.

Mental Acuity. Many women report feeling as if they were living in a fog during their PMS days, forgetfulness and fuzzy thinking being their main complaints. Leaves from the gingko tree, the oldest-surviving tree on earth, have been used to increase memory and reaction time by improving blood flow to the brain.

Gingko is not available as a bulk herb but is available in pill form. This is one instance in which the commercial preparation is preferable because it takes far too many gingko leaves to make medicinal tea practical. If you want sharper mental functioning during PMS days, try one of the commercial preparations available through one of the sources in the Resource List in the back of the book.

Anxiety. As with bloating, there are many herbs available to help with anxiety. Some of those having a sedative or tranquilizing effect are catnip, celery seed, passionflower, hop, skullcap, wild cherry, yarrow, balm, chamomile, and fenugreek. One of the best sedatives is valerian.

Valerian has been used since at least the thirteenth century as a sedative. In 1981 researchers discovered several water-soluble chemicals with apparent sedative properties in valerian, and some have since compared valerian to the pharmaceutical drug Valium. Valerian is, however, a much milder and safer sedative than Valium.

—Although a psychological dependence may develop, valerian is not addictive, and there are no withdrawal symptoms when it is stopped.

—Valerian's sedative effect is not exaggerated by alcohol and barbiturates, as is Valium's.

—Recommended amounts of valerian do not cause morning grogginess, as does Valium.

—Valerian has not been related to birth defects, as has Valium.

For a sedative infusion, steep two teaspoons of powdered root per cup of water for ten to fifteen minutes. Drink one cup before bed. Sweeten with honey or sugar to improve the flavor.

In a tincture take one-half to one teaspoon before bed.

Large doses of valerian can cause headache, giddiness, blurred vision, restlessness, nausea, and morning grogginess.

MORE ALTERNATIVES

Other therapies, some of which come to us from other cultures, have helped many women with PMS symptoms. Although each of these is physically based, many women for whom they work report that they help with psychological symptoms too.

Acupressure, Acupuncture. Ancient Chinese healing practices are still used in many parts of the world. Traditional Oriental medicine sees the body as flowing with chi, or a kind of life energy that Westerners might compare with electromagnetic energy. When the life energy is equally distributed throughout the body in sufficient amounts, a state of health exists.

It is believed that the life energy flows through the body in predictable ways, on paths called meridians. In some places the meridians move deeply, through major organs; in others they run along the surface of the skin. When the energy path is broken or blocked, disease is manifested in the organs the meridian contacts. Then the broken or blocked flow of energy can be corrected by stimulating specific points at the surface meridian locations by inserting hair-thin needles (acupuncture) or by exerting finger or hand pressure (acupressure).

If you are interested in using acupuncture for your PMS symptoms, you need to find a qualified practitioner who understands not only acupuncture but PMS. Some places to look are included in the Resource List. Acupressure can be performed by yourself or by a friend, and the best way to learn it is to take a class or to receive some instruction through charts and books, since it helps to see the points and have specific information on how hard and for how long to apply pressure.

Acupressure has been used to relieve psychological PMS symptoms like anxiety, irritability, mood swings, and depression as well as to help with physical symptoms such as acne, breast tenderness, bloating, fatigue, and headache.

Biofeedback. Because many PMS symptoms are intensified by stress, a therapy that teaches you how to release tension when under stress can be particularly helpful.

The word *biofeedback* describes exactly what this therapy does: It gives you information (feedback) about your biology or physiology (bio). A qualified biofeedback technician can help you to learn your body's signals that tell you:

—when your muscles are tense

—how to notice what you are doing to keep them tense

—how to practice reducing the tension

We all respond to the world on several different levels at one time: emotionally, intellectually, and physically. The three are interrelated. For example, when your boss reads you the riot act or your boyfriend flirts with someone else, whether or not you are aware of it, you respond not only emotionally and intellectually but with subtle changes in your body—mostly in the form of muscle tension. Biofeedback can teach you how to feel and release that tension. You may not have control over your boss's bad days or your boyfriend's wandering eye, but you don't have to pay for them with higher stress levels and intensified PMS symptoms.

Many biofeedback programs are based on two principles: stress management and stress response control.

Stress management teaches you how to identify and handle specific stressors in your life. For example, you may find that you need to learn how to express rather than repress feelings, how to be constructively assertive rather than destructively aggressive, or how to cope with the demands you make on yourself as well as the demands others make on you.

The *stress response control* part of the program determines how you usually respond physically to stress so that you can then map out a program for change.

Most biofeedback programs use three machines to chart your responses. The electromyograph, or EMG unit, measures electrical energy produced by your muscles. Electrodes placed on your skin transmit the strength of the signals; the higher the signal, the higher the tension level.

The second machine, the temperature unit, is a sensor that attaches to the longest finger of your dominant hand. It produces signals you can see and hear in response to your skin temperature.

The third machine is the electrodermal response (EDR) unit. It measures the sweat gland's response to stress. Most people sweat more when they are under stress, sometimes in amounts so small you wouldn't notice without the machine. Sweat-covered skin conducts electricity more easily than does dry skin, so a small amount of electrical current is passed through your skin between two electrodes to measure the conductivity. Higher conductivity means more sweat and a higher level of stress. Like the readouts from the other machines described here, those from the EDR can help you recognize a stress response even when that response may not be noticeable by everyday physical standards.

Since being able to relax under stress is one of the goals of biofeedback, some programs teach you how to use relaxation tapes so that you can practice the techniques outside the lab too.

Of course, there's no magic in the machines; they are simply tools that can help you become more aware of certain facts about your physiological functioning that you wouldn't easily know otherwise. A good biofeedback technician guides you through the learning process, but the responsibility lies with you to practice the techniques you learn in the lab. Many women see biofeedback training as a personal resource that allows them control over their reactions to difficult situations they cannot change.

If you are interested in trying biofeedback methods for controlling some of your responses to PMS and the stress that can make it worse, ask your physician for a referral, or contact the source listed in the Resource List.

Yoga. Many women have found help for some of their PMS symptoms through practicing yoga exercises. The traditional goal of yoga, which was developed about five thousand years ago in India, has been to promote harmony and balance in the practitioner. When it is done properly, yoga practice has a healthy effect on many levels: physical, mental, emotional, and spiritual.

Hatha-yoga, the type most commonly taught in the United States, is based on physical exercises or postures called asanas and breathing exercises called *pranauama*.

Community centers, recreation centers, and YWCAs everywhere offer yoga classes. Check your local sources for a class.

WHAT *NOT* TO DO FOR PMS

This book outlines scores of ways to relieve PMS symptoms. Many of them have worked at least to some degree for thousands of women. But there are a few cautions to keep in mind. Be wary of:

—"instant" cures for PMS. An instant cure can be an unrealistic promise from an unqualified counselor or your own belief that if you just eat a perfectly balanced diet, all your PMS symptoms will disappear. Because no one has identified a single clear cause for PMS, there is no single instant cure. But there are lots of things you can do that help.

—unnecessary diagnostic procedures. If someone tells you that you need an expensive round of "hormone testing" or high-tech assessment tools to determine if you have PMS (not to rule out another condition), find a different health care provider. The only way to diagnose PMS is through charting your symptoms.

—long-term psychoactive drug treatment when you do not have an underlying psychological disorder. While some of these drugs have helped some women in the short term, medical sources agree that without an underlying psychological problem, taking these kinds of drugs over long periods of time is not helpful.

—long-term diuretic use. Because no studies have shown that these seriously help PMS symptoms, their long-term use may cause more problems than they are worth.

SEVEN

DEVELOPING YOUR PERSONAL PMS PHILOSOPHY

An important question that may have occurred to you as you have read through this book is: What, after all, is the goal of PMS treatment? Should you *always* feel calm, smooth, harmonious—no ruffled feathers, loud voices, wild rages no matter what time of the month it is? Further, is PMS treatment intended to *fix* a disorder? Are you ill or do you have a disease if you have PMS?

There are no easy answers to these questions. In fact, they fuel the controversy that often surrounds PMS and its research in medical and lay circles alike.

So far this book has focused on conventional and alternative treatments you might choose to help change how you feel—physically and emotionally—in the days before your period. This chapter will examine another approach: that of seeing PMS and your menstrual cycle as a whole in a *positive* light.

ANOTHER VIEW

There are those who claim that calling PMS a disorder is the same as calling menopause a disease or pregnancy an illness. While this view does not deny the physical realities of how you may feel a week or two before your period, it does say that even if you find yourself on an emotional roller coaster, that may not be all bad.

For example, some anthropologists have started to ask why it is that only Western cultures report PMS as a problem. One theory is that our industrialized society requires of its workers a certain kind of discipline: We bend our ways to fulfill workplace requirements rather than change how we do our work to fit what we need in our personal lives. So, do women who have more required of them—in the office or at home—experience more intense PMS symptoms? The answer is yes, in many cases. More stress, no matter where it comes from, means more PMS. And some studies show that the incidence of PMS increases with each of these stress-producing factors: age, number of children, and the presence of a male living partner.

The same anthropologists posing these questions theorize that this is not a major area of investigation because in societies like ours, it's unthinkable that the inflexibility of the *society* could be the problem that needs fixing. Instead, we see the *women* as malfunctioning and in need of having their "hormonal imbalances" fixed.

It's not likely that society will be transformed anytime soon, but you can transform how you see your own PMS time. Maybe you don't fit into your demanding life as smoothly as you do at other times of the month, but during those days perhaps you could see that:

—your loss of concentration and focus equals a gain in creativity and the ability to free-associate

—your loss of muscle control and your "clumsiness" equal an incredible ability to relax

—your decreased efficiency equals an ability to give increased attention to a smaller number of tasks

—your depression and melancholy equal a monthly opportunity to reflect and pull inward to see what's *really* going on inside you

—your increased crying equals an increase in feeling and expression

In all, you can choose to see your PMS time as a time of increased capacity for emotional responsiveness, sensitivity, and creativity. Perhaps the *real* issue is that there is no convenient space for these elemental parts of yourself in the workaday world and that during your PMS time—arguably your most elemental time—these hidden abilities and feelings are so strong they simply can't be restrained.

UNDERSTANDING ANGER

Many women are most bothered by the anger that rages out of them at PMS times. In our culture it is primarily the woman's job to see that social relationships, family ties, and love all run smoothly. If a woman is angry, she disrupts the family or upsets those around her and sets in motion a cycle, one that runs from disruption to guilt to depression over not keeping peace wherever she is and over allowing her feelings to intrude upon others.

Some sociologists believe that women aren't actually more angry on PMS days. Rather, during that time women tend to ignore the internal censors that normally stop them from expressing anger. Annoyances you put up with at other times of the month suddenly seem ridiculous and unbearable, and you may be more likely to act on or express your anger.

The question usually asked is: "How can I keep my temper under control during my PMS time?" Maybe the question also needs to be: "How can I learn from those rages?" You may be able to answer both if you write your rages in a journal and read those words at a calmer time. Esther Rome, a coauthor of *The New Our Bodies, Ourselves,* says that "calling these times of rage symptoms of disease is a handy way of not looking at what women are upset about and why."

KEEPING A JOURNAL

For some women keeping a journal is the most helpful tool in understanding themselves. Your journal may tell you more about your PMS times than you could have guessed; journals often have a way of revealing unexpected truths.

A journal may be anything. If you are at work, notes in your Day-Timer, on your calendar, or on your computer can constitute a journal. Or you might have a special notebook reserved for PMS days. Journals are similar to diaries, but the focus is on inner thoughts and feelings rather than external events. That's why they work so well for some people; the act of recording thoughts and feelings forces the writer to slow down and analyze what's going on inside herself.

For many people who keep journals, it is the most difficult aspects of their lives that are recorded; the journal becomes the companion in troubled times as well as the place where the most painful feelings are worked through. If you have particularly rocky emotional times during your PMS days, you may find that writing them in a journal is especially helpful. Some women also feel that writing down their rages keeps them from visiting them unfairly on others.

There are now nearly two dozen books on the market that can help you get started with journal keeping. If you want to get started right away, here are some tips from journal therapist Kathleen Adams, who wrote *Journal to the Self: Twenty-two Paths to Personal Growth:*

—Relax. Take a few deep breaths and shift into neutral before you begin.

—Date every entry. This allows you to notice cycles and trends in your life.

—Keep what you write. Even entries that seem to be junk can be useful.

—Write quickly. This increases spontaneity and reduces writer's block.

—Start writing and keep writing. This guards against interrupting your flow of thought.

—Tell the complete truth quickly. Get to the bottom line, and don't pretend you don't know what's going on when you do.

—Protect your privacy. Keep your journal in a safe place.

—Write naturally. In journal writing there are no rules. Write in a way that feels comfortable and real.

TRACKING YOUR DREAMS

Your dreams might also help you explore premenstrual emotions. Some studies suggest that the amount women dream, as well as how much they recall of their dreams, varies with the stage of their menstrual cycle and how much estrogen is being produced. Some investigators have reported that the peak of dreaming and recall occurs between ovulation (when estrogen is high) and the onset of menstruation (when estrogen is low). Some have also reported that postmenopausal women who take estrogen to replace their own dream more than those who don't.

Whatever the exact connection between hormones and dreaming, more than one researcher has found that women have an increased need to dream premenstrually and that they are most likely to dream more when they feel the irritability, depression, and fatigue of PMS. Their studies have shown that women without PMS symptoms tend to *sleep* more right before their periods; women with PMS tend to *dream* more then.

Many people, psychologists and dream therapists among them, believe that dreams give us direct access to the subconscious. If you would like to tap into this resource to help you understand and learn from your PMS times, you might like to read *Women's Bodies, Women's Dreams,* by Patricia Garfield, Ph.D. She suggests these steps to begin recording your dreams:

—Set aside a special journal for dream entries.

—Each evening write a brief note about what happened that day, especially your feelings about the events.

—Put a notepad and pencil beside your bed before going to sleep. During the night, if you awaken, or in the morning, jot down key words and phrases from any dreams.

—When you have time during the day or before going to bed the next night, write a description of your dreams of the previous night.

Garfield indicates that by using her system of dream images as an interpretation tool, you can begin to understand what your PMS dreams may be telling you.

One characteristic of PMS dreams, according to Garfield, is increased creativity. In fact, many women report a surge of creativity just before and/or during their periods, and Garfield speculates that an inward focus during those days brings a sharper awareness of that creativity and ways to use it. She adds: "Women often speak of being 'spacey' and having difficulty focusing on details on PMS days. The positive side of this condition is that it is easier to free-associate, to come up with new combinations of familiar things in unfamiliar ways—this is what constitutes creativity."

CREATING A MOON LODGE

Some Native American cultures characterize PMS days as having particular strength, wisdom, and insight, a belief deeply rooted in a spiritual and cultural heritage still practiced. Anthropologists are beginning to see they were mistaken in their earlier interpretations of menstrual practices in some traditional cultures as signs of "uncleanness" and taboo. Instead, they now understand that often the isolation of premenstrual or menstruating women was a form of honor rather than shame.

For example, some Yurok women, Native Americans still living on their ancestral lands in northwestern California, have resurrected traditional menstrual and premenstrual practices taught them by aunts and grandmothers. As one Yurok woman described it, during her PMS time a woman should "isolate herself because this is the time when she is at the height of her powers. Thus the time should not be wasted in mundane tasks and social distractions, nor should one's concentration be broken by concerns with the opposite sex." Instead, all of a woman's energies should be applied in meditation "to find out the purpose of your life" and toward the "accumulation" of spiritual energy.

Traditionally women shared these days just before and during their periods in dome-shaped brush lodges, away from regular chores and men. Today Yurok women may have small rooms in their homes that they use for their retreat or sheds or huts built on their land for this purpose, or they may simply camp with other women for these days.

Many non–Native American women also see value in this monthly retreat. While it's not possible for most women to disappear from their families, male friends, and spouses for several days each month (as tantalizing as that may seem), you can create a regular breathing space to help ease yourself through your most difficult PMS days.

One way to do that is to participate in a moon lodge. While this approach is not for everyone, several women around the country offer moon lodge retreats. Some of those running these retreats are Native Americans; some are midwives; some are psychologists and psychotherapists. Two moon lodge retreats are included in the Resource List.

If participating in someone else's moon lodge doesn't

seem to be a possibility for you, you could set up your own moon lodge ritual. Carole Shane, a midwife who with psychotherapist Christina Nealson offers a moon lodge, believes that creating one for yourself honors who you are biologically in ways our culture doesn't. Shane points to the language sometimes used to describe PMS behavior: It's "only" my hormones, or it's "just" my period. In every way, from language to actions, she says, we diminish the importance of cycles that are an intimate part of who we are.

Tips on how to create your own moon lodge:

—Take time to *be alone* and feel the feelings you have—positive or negative. Shane believes the days around your period are highly spiritual, the perfect time for a "vision quest" in which you seek wisdom and knowledge.

—*Protect* yourself, because you may be at your most emotionally vulnerable during your PMS time. Shane believes the uterus, so intimately involved with menstruation, is physically and emotionally the most receptive organ in women's bodies, the place where they are most likely to receive and hold hurts and fears. Protecting yourself in this case means not scheduling for this time meetings you know will be especially difficult or threatening. Don't attempt to solo with your children on outings you know will stress you beyond your limits. Don't put additional requirements on yourself.

You can figure out when to schedule your time alone (a whole day or just a few hours) by charting your cycles as described in Chapter 3.

How will you spend your time alone? Some ideas from Shane:

—Sit quietly.

—Sleep.

—Pray or meditate.

—Write in a special journal.

—Spend the time doing whatever turns you inward.

PUTTING IT ALL TOGETHER

You now have the tools to understand and find relief from your PMS symptoms. Keep in mind that because there is no single cause of PMS, no one remedy will likely erase all your symptoms. But you have taken a big step in the right direction by gaining a more specific understanding of your body and its cycles, by consulting with a physician, and by simply trying approaches explained in this book until you find ones that work for you.

GLOSSARY

Basal body temperature (BBT) chart: A chart used to graph daily basal temperature (upon awakening and before any activity) during the menstrual cycle to discern when ovulation takes place.

Beta-endorphins: One of a family of polypeptides (amino acids) found in the brain that have the same effect as an opiate and can induce feelings of well-being and act as a pain-killer.

Cervix: A fibrous ring of tissue joining the uterus to the vagina.

Corpus luteum: Means "yellow body." After ovulation the empty follicle becomes a gland called the corpus luteum, which produces progesterone to prepare the endometrial lining of the uterus for implantation by a fertilized egg, or embryo.

Dysmenorrhea: Painful menstrual periods.

Endometriosis: A condition in which endometrial tissue (normal uterine lining) is implanted in abnormal places outside the uterus, grows, and bleeds or becomes inflamed during the menstrual cycle. Sometimes PMS is misdiagnosed as endometriosis.

Endometrium: The mucous membrane that lines the uterus. It either nurtures the implanted embryo or is expelled during a menstrual period.

Estrogen: The primary female hormone, produced mainly in the ovaries from puberty to menopause. Produced by the developing egg follicle, it stimulates the enrichment of the uterine lining for implantation of an embryo and causes changes in cervical mucus that indicate ovulation is imminent.

Fallopian tubes: Also called oviducts. Two sturdy tubes, each about four inches long, that rise from the top of the uterus on either side to the ovaries. After the release of an egg from the ovary, the egg is transported down the tube to the uterus.

Follicular phase: The first phase of the menstrual cycle during which follicles develop from Day 1 to about Day 13 of the cycle.

Gonadotropin-releasing hormone (GnRH): The hormone secreted by the hypothalamus that signals the pituitary to release follicle-stimulating hormone and luteinizing hormone.

Hypoglycemia: Low blood sugar caused by abnormal function of the pancreas. Sometimes confused with PMS because it may have similar symptoms.

Hypothalamus: An area of the brain near the pituitary that controls hormonal secretions of the pituitary.

Hysterectomy: A surgical procedure in which all or part of the uterus is removed.

Luteal phase: The third part of the menstrual cycle, after ovulation, in which progesterone is produced by the corpus luteum to prepare the endometrium for implantation of a fertilized egg. During this phase PMS symptoms occur.

Menarche: The first menstrual period in a girl's life, usually occurring around the age of eleven or twelve in the United States.

Menopause: The cessation of menstruation. Usually occurs around age fifty-one in the United States.

Menstrual cycle: The monthly cycle of ovulation, usually twenty-five to thirty-five days long, counted from the first day of the menstrual period.

Menstrual period: The fourth phase of the menstrual cycle in which, when there is no pregnancy, the endometrial lining of the uterus is shed, producing menstrual bleeding.

Ovary: Female reproductive organ that stores and releases eggs and produces the hormones estrogen and progesterone. There are two ovaries, located on either side of the uterus and connected to it by a thin stalk, slightly behind the Fallopian tubes.

Pituitary: An endocrine gland located near the base of the brain that secretes hormones and coordinates the message system that supports the menstrual cycle.

Progesterone: A female hormone produced by the ovaries in the second or luteal phase of the cycle.

Prostaglandins: Chemicals produced by the lining of the uterus, increasing until menstruation. Some research has shown they are partly responsible for menstrual cramps and may be implicated in some PMS symptoms.

Tubal ligation: A surgical procedure in which the Fallopian tubes are severed and/or sealed to prevent pregnancy.

Uterus: The hollow pear-shaped muscular organ in which a fetus is implanted and nurtured until birth. If there is no pregnancy, the lining of the uterus, built up each month

during the menstrual cycle, is shed during a menstrual
period.

Vagina: The muscular passage between the vulva and the
cervix through which menstrual fluids pass.

Vulva: Folds of skin that protect the entrance to the vagina.

RESOURCE LIST

ACUPUNCTURE/ACUPRESSURE

Acupuncture International Association
2330 South Brentwood Boulevard
St. Louis, Missouri 63144
314-961-2300
Doctors, chiropractors, and osteopaths who practice acupuncture.

American Association for Acupuncture and
   Oriental Medicine
1424 Sixteenth Street NW, Suite 501
Washington, D.C. 20036
202-265-2287

California Certified Acupuncturists Association
259 Eighth Street, Suite 202
Oakland, California 94607
415-444-3868
Will refer to local California areas or for specific need.
(Check your local telephone directory for state associations

of certified acupuncturists. These specialists usually also
know acupressure.)

California Acupuncture Association
2180 Garnet Avenue, No. 3G-1
San Diego, California 92109
619-270-1005
Acts as a referral service for acupuncturists, some of whom
are trained in the use of herbal treatments.

BIOFEEDBACK

Association for Applied Psychophysiology and Biofeedback
c/o Francine Butler, Ph.D.
10200 West Forty-fourth Street, No. 304
Wheatridge, Colorado 80033
303-422-8436

HERBALISTS

American Herbalists Guild
Box 1683
Soquel, California 95073
Provides lists of courses and educational programs in the
use of herbs. Sponsors annual symposium. Will answer
herb-related questions but is not a referral service.

American Association of Naturopathic Physicians
Box 20386
Seattle, Washington 98102
206-323-7610

Acts as a referral service for naturopathic physicians who practice holistic treatment methods.

BULK HERBS, TINCTURES, OILS, AND TABLETS

The Herb and Spice Collection
Box 118
Norway, Iowa 52318
Free catalog includes 150 medicinal herbs.

HerbPharm's Whole Herb Catalog
Box 116
Williams, Oregon 97544
503-846-6262
Free catalog of 100 herb oils and more.

Nature's Herbs
1010 Forty-sixth Street
Emeryville, California 94608
510-601-0700
Free catalog of 350 herbs and spices.

NUTRITIONALLY ORIENTED HEALTH CARE

American Dietitians Association
216 West Jackson Boulevard, Suite 800
Chicago, Illinois 60606
312-899-0040

Will answer questions on nutrition over the telephone. Offers list of consulting dieticians by state.

Prevention Magazine Reader's Service
Emmaus, Pennsylvania 18049
215-967-8038
Indexes articles by subject from *Prevention* magazine and related newsletters published by Rodale Press. Will supply copies in response to telephone or mail queries.

ORGANIZATIONS, CLINICS, AND PHYSICIANS OFFERING PMS SERVICES

PMS Treatment Center
Box 20998, Dept. PN
Portland, Oregon 97220
Offers psychological, medical, and life-style evaluation and treatments for PMS by physicians, psychologists, and counselors on staff. Has also compiled a PMS physician referral list. To receive it, send five dollars and a stamped (two twenty-nine-cent stamps), self-addressed business-size envelope for an educational packet and a list of doctors in your area who specialize in treating PMS. Physicians and counselors from this center will travel to other parts of the country to assist health care professionals in establishing their own PMS clinics and will speak to professional and community groups on PMS topics.

National Women's Health Network
1325 G Street NW
Washington, D.C. 20005
202-347-1140

National public interest organization focusing on women's health issues. Write or call for information packet ($5) on PMS, along with list of recommended reading.

PMS Access
Box 9326
Madison, Wisconsin 53715
800-222-4PMS (4767)
Wisconsin: call 608-833-4PMS; 9:00 A.M. to 5:00 P.M., central time, Monday to Friday
A division of Madison Pharmacy Associates, which produces PMS products. It provides an information line offering a free packet of self-help information. You can order a doctor referral list within your zip code area for $9.95 plus shipping and handling. PMS Access also publishes a quarterly newsletter and maintains a library that sells PMS books.

PMS Clinic
1800 Thirtieth Street, Suite 308
Boulder, Colorado 80301
303-440-7100
Offers a range of services from counseling, help with diet, and exercise treatments to medical treatments.

PMS Self-Help Center
170 State Street, Suite 222
Los Altos, California 94022
415-964-7268
Provides educational materials about PMS, seminars, workshops, and treatment.

OTHER ALTERNATIVES

Alternative Medicine Foundation
Dr. Donald G. DeLong
4519 Admiralty Way, Suite 201
Marina Del Rey, California 90292
213-823-6355
Clinical psychologist trained in marriage, family, and child counseling uses regression therapy to treat emotional aspects of PMS. Works in concert with endocrinologist as needed.

MOON LODGE WORKSHOPS

Carole Shane and Christina Nealson
4396 Snowberry Court
Boulder, Colorado 80304
303-440-4146

Brooke Medicine Eagle
P.O. Box 1682
Helena, Montana 59624

BOOKS FOR MORE INFORMATION

Castleman, Michael. *The Healing Herbs: The Ultimate Guide to the Curative Power of Nature's Medicine.* Emmaus, Pa.: Rodale Press, 1991. The definitive herb book covering a hundred healing herbs, including their uses, safe dosages, and preparation.

Francia, Luisa. *Dragontime: Magic and Mystery of Men-*

struation. Woodstock, N.Y.: Ash Tree Publishing, 1991. An alternative, positive look at menstruation and all that goes with it, including PMS.

Garfield, Patricia, Ph.D. *Women's Bodies, Women's Dreams.* New York: Ballantine, 1988. A hands-on, comprehensive guide to understanding how women's dreams reflect and lend insight to their bodily changes.

Graedon, Joe. *The People's Pharmacy: Totally New and Revised.* New York: St. Martin's Press, 1985. Guide to prescription and nonprescription drugs.

Griffith, H. Winter, M.D. *Complete Guide to Prescription and Non-prescription Drugs. Complete Guide to Vitamins, Minerals and Supplements.* Tucson, Arizona: H.P. Books, 1991. Good sources for checking on uses and side effects of drugs and vitamins.

Mindell, Earl. *Earl Mindell's New and Revised Vitamin Bible.* New York: Warner Books, 1985. A complete listing of vitamins and other nutrients (minerals, proteins, fats) and their uses.

Shannon, Marilyn. *Fertility, Cycles and Nutrition.* Cincinnati: Couple to Couple League. Specific nutritional approaches for relief from PMS symptoms.

Taylor, Dena. *Red Flower: Rethinking Menstruation.* Freedom, Calif.: Crossing Press, 1988. Debunks myths and prejudices surrounding menstruation, including PMS.

BIBLIOGRAPHY

BOOKS

Adams, Kathleen. *Journal to the Self: Twenty-two Steps to Personal Growth.* New York: Warner Books, 1990.

Bender, Stephanie DeGraff, M.A. *PMS: A Positive Program to Gain Control.* Tucson, Arizona. Body Press, 1986.

Berger, Gilda. *PMS: Premenstrual Syndrome.* New York: Franklin Watts, 1984.

Boston Women's Health Collective. *The New Our Bodies, Ourselves.* New York: Simon & Schuster, 1984.

Buckley, Thomas, and Alma Gottlieb, eds. *Blood Magic: The Anthropology of Menstruation.* Berkeley: University of California Press, 1988.

Castleman, Michael. *The Healing Herbs.* Emmaus, Pa.: Rodale Press, 1991.

Dalton, Katharina. *Once a Month.* Claremont, Calif.: Hunter House, 1983.

Dawood, M. Yusoff, M.D., et al. *Premenstrual Syndrome and Dysmenorrhea.* Baltimore-Munich: Urban & Schwarzenberg, 1985.

Delaney, Janice, et al. *The Curse: A Cultural History of Menstruation.* New York: E. P. Dutton & Co., 1976.

Demmers, Laurence M., Ph.D. et al., eds. *Premenstrual, Postpartum, and Menopausal Mood Disorders.* Baltimore-Munich: Urban & Schwarzenberg, 1989.

Francia, Luisa. *Dragontime: Magic and Mystery of Menstruation.* Woodstock, N.Y.: Ash Tree Press, 1991.

Gannon, Linda R. *Menstrual Disorders and Menopause: Biological, Psychological and Cultural Research.* New York: Praeger Publishers, 1985.

Garfield, Patricia, Ph.D. *Women's Bodies, Women's Dreams.* New York: Ballantine, 1988.

Halas, Celia, Ph.D. *Relief from Premenstrual Syndrome.* New York: Frederick Fell Publishers, 1984.

Harrison, Michelle. *Self-Help for Premenstrual Syndrome.* New York: Random House, 1985.

Hughes, Martin, M.D. *Body Clock: Effects of Time on Human Health.* Oxford: Facts on File, 1988.

Lander, Louise. *Images of Bleeding: Menstruation as Ideology.* New York: Orlando Press, 1988.

Lark, Susan M., M.D. *Dr. Susan Lark's Premenstrual Syndrome Self-Help Book: A Woman's Guide to Feeling Good All Month.* Los Angeles: Forman Publishing, 1984.

Lever, Judy. *Pre-Menstrual Tension.* New York: Bantam, 1982.

Magalini, Sergio L., and Euclide Scrascia. *Dictionary of Medical Syndromes,* 2d ed. Philadelphia: J. B. Lippincott Co., 1981.

Mindell, Earl. *Earl Mindell's New and Revised Vitamin Bible.* New York: Warner Books, 1985.

Norris, Ronald V., M.D. *PMS: Premenstrual Syndrome.* New York: Rawson Associates, 1983.

Olesen, Virginia L., and Nancy Fugate Woods, eds. *Culture, Society, and Menstruation.* New York: Hemisphere Publishing Corp., 1986.

Schneider, Carol J., Ph.D., and Edgar S. Wilson, M.D. *Foun-

dations of Biofeedback Practice. Denver: Biofeedback Society of America. 1985.

Schwartz, Mark S., and Assoc. *Biofeedback: A Practitioner's Guide*. New York: Guilford Press, 1987.

Severino, Sally K., M.D., and Margaret L. Moline, Ph.D. *Premenstrual Syndrome: A Clinician's Guide*. New York: Guilford Press, 1989.

Shuttle, Penelope, and Peter Redgrove. *The Wise Wound: Myths, Realities and Meanings of Menstruation*. New York: Bantam, 1990.

Stoppard, Miriam, M.D. *Everywoman's Medical Handbook*. New York: Ballantine, 1988.

Taylor, Dena. *Red Flower: Rethinking Menstruation*. Freedom, Calif.: Crossing Press, 1988.

Weideger, Paula. *Menstruation and Menopause: The Physiology and Psychology, the Myth and the Reality*. New York: Alfred A. Knopf, 1976.

ARTICLES, JOURNALS, NEWSLETTERS

———. "Breaking Attitude Stereotypes." *USA Today*, February, 1989.

———. "PMS from a Feminist Perspective." *PMS Access*, no. 32 (July–August 1990).

———. "Self-Esteem: Public and Private Policies." *PMS Access*, no. 30 (March–April 1990).

———. "PMS Eased by Vitamin E." *Prevention* (December 1987).

———. "PMS Study Pans Popular Prescription." *Science News* (July 21, 1990).

———. "PMS-Related Depression." *PMS Access*, no. 25 (May–June 1989).

————. "Review of Gonadotropin-Releasing Hormone Agonist Study." *PMS Access*, no. 1 (May–June 1985).

————. "Progesterone: The Hormone, the Medication." *PMS Access*, no. 23 (January–February 1989).

————. "PMS Software Developed." *PMS Access*, no. 25 (May–June 1989).

————. "Hysterectomy and Tubal Ligation: PMS Cause or Treatment?" *PMS Access*, no. 27 (September–October 1990).

————. "PMS and Thyroid Dysfunction." *PMS Access*, no. 13 (May–June 1987).

————. "PMS and Candida Albican Yeast Theory." *PMS Access*, no. 10 (November–December 1986).

————. "The PMS Movement: Exercise as Therapy." *PMS Access*, no. 5 (January–February 1986).

————. "Amino Acids: A Link to PMS." *PMS Access*, no. 6 (March–April 1986).

————. "The Race to Reduce Stress." *PMS Access*, no. 29 (January–February 1990).

————. "Chase Away Premenstrual Blues." *Redbook* (September 1990).

————. "Hypoglycemia: Low Blood Sugar Linked to Physical and Emotional Woe." *PMS Access*, no. 22 (November–December 1988).

————. "PMS and Panic Disorders." *PMS Access*, no. 17 (January–February 1988).

————. "Sick and Tired: Struggling with Chronic Epstein-Barr Virus." *PMS Access*, no. 18 (March–April 1988).

————. "PMS Pill." *Prevention* (February 1989).

————. "Old Problem, New 'Disease': The Controversy Surrounding PMS." *National Women's Health Network* (Summer 1984).

————. "PMS and the Working Woman." *PMS Access*, no. 4 (November–December 1985).

————. "PMS and the Family." *PMS Access,* no. 3 (September–October 1985).

Ainscough, C. E. "Premenstrual Emotional Changes: A Prospective Study of Symptomatology in Normal Women." *Journal of Psychosomatic Residency,* vol. 34, no. 1 (1990).

Bains, G. K., and P. Slade. "Attributional Patterns, Moods and the Menstrual Cycle." *Psychosomatic Medicine,* vol. 50, no. 5 (September–October 1988).

Bender, Stephanie DeGraff, M.A. "PMS Recovery: What's Next?" *PMS Access,* no. 32 (July–August 1990).

Berman, M. K., et al. "Vitamin B_6 in Premenstrual Syndrome." *Journal of the American Dietetic Association,* vol. 90, no. 6 (June 1990).

Boyd, N. F., et al. "Effect of a Low-Fat High-Carbohydrate Diet on Symptoms of Cyclical Mastopathy." *Lancet,* vol. 2, no. 8603 (July 16, 1988).

Brown, S., et al. "The Influence of Method of Contraception and Cigarette Smoking on Menstrual Patterns." *British Journal of Obstetrics and Gynecology,* vol. 95, no. 9 (September 1988).

Brush, M. G., et al. "Pyridoxine in the Treatment of Premenstrual Syndrome: A Retrospective Survey in 630 Patients." *British Journal of Clinical Practice,* vol. 42, no. 11 (November 1988).

Brzezinski, A. A., et al. "D-Fenfluramine Suppresses the Increased Calorie and Carbohydrate Intakes and Improves the Mood of Women with Premenstrual Depression." *Obstetrics and Gynecology,* vol. 76, no. 2 (August 1990).

Busch, C. M., et al. "Severe Perimenstrual Symptoms: Prevalence and Effects on Absenteeism and Health Care Seeking in a Non-Clinical Sample." *Women Health,* vol. 14, no. 1 (1988).

Cameron, O. G., et al. "Menstrual Fluctuation in the Symptoms of Panic Anxiety." *Journal of Affective Disorders,* vol. 15, no. 2 (September–October 1988).

Casper, R. F., and M. T. Hearn. "The Effect of Hysterectomy and Bilateral Oophorectomy in Women with Severe Premenstrual Syndrome." *American Journal of Obstetrics and Gynecology,* vol. 162, no. 1 (January 1990).

Casson, P., et al. "Lasting Response to Ovariectomy in Severe Intractable Premenstrual Syndrome." *American Journal of Obstetrics and Gynecology,* vol. 162, no. 1 (January 1990).

Chuong, C. J., et al. "Clinical Trial of Naltrexone in Premenstrual Syndrome." *Obstetrics and Gynecology,* vol. 72, no. 3 (September 1988).

Chrisler, J. C., and K. B. Levy. "The Media Construct a Menstrual Monster: A Content Analysis of PMS Articles in the Popular Press." *Women Health,* vol. 16, no. 2 (1990).

Christensen, A. P., and T. P. Oei. "Men's Perception of Premenstrual Changes on the Premenstrual Assessment Form." *Psychology Rep.,* vol. 66, no. 2 (April 1990).

Clementz, G. L., and J. W. Dailey. "Psychotropic Effects of Caffeine." *American Family Physician,* vol. 37, no. 5 (May 1988).

Cortese, J., and M. A. Brown. "Coping Responses of Men Whose Partners Experience Premenstrual Symptomatology." *Journal of Obstetrical Gynecological and Neonatal Nursing,* vol. 18, no. 5 (September–October 1989).

Coupey, S. M., and P. Ahlstrom. "Common Menstrual Disorders." *Pediatric Clinician of North America,* vol. 36, no. 3 (June 1989).

Denicoff, K. D., et al. "Glucose Tolerance Testing in Women with Premenstrual Syndrome." *American Journal of Psychiatry,* vol. 147, no. 4 (April 1990).

Denning, D. W., et al. "The Relationship Between Normal Fluid Retention in Women and Idiopathic Oedema." *Postgraduate Medical Journal,* vol. 66, no. 775 (May 1990).

Derzko, C. M. "Role of Danazol in Relieving the Premenstrual Syndrome." *Journal of Reproductive Medicine,* vol. 35, no. 1 (supplement) (January 1990).

Devalon, M. S., and J. W. Bachman. "Premenstrual Syndrome. A Practical Approach to Management." *Postgraduate Medicine,* vol. 86, no. 7 (November 15, 1989).

Doll, H., et al. "Pyridoxine and the Premenstrual Syndrome: A Randomized Crossover Trial." *Journal of the Royal College of General Practitioners,* vol. 39, no. 326 (September 1989).

Dranov, Paula. "An Unkind Cut." *American Health,* vol. 9, no. 7 (September 1990).

Endicott, J., and U. Halbreich. "Clinical Significance of Premenstrual Dysphoric Changes." *Journal of Clinical Psychiatry,* vol. 49, no. 12 (December 1988).

Ensign, J. E., et al. "Premenstrual Syndrome: Etiology and Treatment Possibilities." *AORN Journal,* vol. 47, no. 4 (April 1988).

Eriksson, E., et al. "Effect of Clomipramine on Premenstrual Syndrome." *Acta Psychiatria Scandinavia,* vol. 81, no. 1 (January 1990).

Facchinetti, F., et al. "Naproxen Sodium in the Treatment of Premenstrual Symptoms." *Gynecological and Obstetrical Investigations,* vol. 28, no. 4 (1989).

Fackelmann, K. A. "PMS: Hints of a Link to Lunchtime and Zinc." *Science News* (October 27, 1990).

Fisher, M., et al. "Premenstrual Symptoms in Adolescents." *Journal of Adolescent Health Care,* vol. 10, no. 5 (September 1989).

Freeman, D. W., et al. "Effects of Medical History Factors

on Symptom Severity in Women Meeting Criteria for Premenstrual Syndrome." *Obstetrics and Gynecology,* vol. 72, no. 2 (August 1988).

Freeman, E., et al. "The Ineffectiveness of Progesterone Suppository Treatment for Premenstrual Syndrome." *Journal of the American Medical Association,* vol. 264, no. 3 (July 18, 1990).

Gannon, L., et al. "Perimenstrual Symptoms: Relationships with Chronic Stress and Selected Lifestyle Variables." *Behavioral Medicine,* vol. 15, no. 4 (Winter 1989).

Gannon, L. "The Potential Role of Exercise in the Alleviation of Menstrual Disorders and Menopausal Symptoms: A Theoretical Synthesis of Recent Research." *Women Health,* vol. 14, no. 2 (1988).

Giannini A. J., et al. "Clonidine in the Treatment of Premenstrual Syndrome: A Subgroup Study." *Journal of Clinical Psychiatry,* vol. 49, no. 2 (February 1988).

Gise, L. H., et al. "Issues in the Identification of Premenstrual Syndromes." *Journal of Nervous and Mental Disorders,* vol. 178, no. 4 (April 1990).

Goodale, I. L., et al. "Alleviation of Premenstrual Syndrome Symptoms with the Relaxation Response." *Obstetrics and Gynecology,* vol. 75, no. 4 (April 1990).

Goodwin, P. J., et al. "Cyclical Mastopathy: A Critical Review of Therapy." *British Journal of Surgery,* vol. 75, no. 9 (September 1988).

Hammarback, S., and T. Backstrom. "Induced Anovulation as Treatment of Premenstrual Tension Syndrome." *Acta Obstetrica Gynecologia of Scandinavia,* vol. 67, no. 2 (1988).

———. "A Demographic Study in Subgroups of Women Seeking Help for Premenstrual Syndrome." *Acta Obstetrica Gynecologia Scandinavia,* vol. 68, no. 3 (1989).

Hammarback S., et al. "Relationship Between Symptom Severity and Hormone Changes in Women with Premenstrual Syndrome." *Journal of Clinical Endocrinology and Metabolism,* vol. 68, no. 1 (January 1989).

Harrison, W. M., et al. "Treatment of Premenstrual Dysphoria with Alprazolam." *Archives of General Psychiatry,* vol. 47, no. 3 (March 1990).

Henig, Robin Marantz. "Dispelling Menstrual Myths." *The New York Times Magazine.* March 7, 1982.

Ho, K. Y., and M. O. Thorner. "Therapeutic Applications of Bromocriptine in Endocrine and Neurological Diseases." *Drugs,* vol. 36, no. 1 (July 1988).

Khoo, S. K., et al. "Evening Primrose Oil and Treatment of Premenstrual Syndrome." *Medical Journal of Australia,* vol. 153, no. 4 (August 20, 1990).

King, C. R. "Parallels Between Neurasthenia and Premenstrual Syndrome." *Women Health,* vol. 15, no. 4, 1989.

Kunes, Ellen. "To the Rescue—the PMS Diet." *Mademoiselle* (March 1990).

Laessle, R. G., et al. "Mood Changes and Physical Complaints During Normal Menstrual Cycle in Healthy Young Women." *Psychoneuroendocrinology,* vol. 15, no. 2 (1990).

Leary, Warren E. "Hopeful Findings for Premenstrual Syndrome." *The New York Times,* December 7, 1989.

———. "Clue Seen to Depression in Premenstrual Women." *The New York Times,* January 8, 1991.

Lippert, Joan. "Easing Monthly Misery." *Ladies' Home Journal* (November 1990).

Lurie, S., and R. Borenstein. "The Premenstrual Syndrome." *Obstetrics and Gynecology Survey,* vol. 45, no. 4 (April 1990).

McFarland, C., et al. "Women's Theories of Menstruation and Biases in Recall of Menstrual Symptoms." *Journal of*

Personal and Social Psychology, vol. 57, no. 3 (September 1989).

Machlin, L. J. "Use and Safety of Elevated Dosages of Vitamin E in Adults." *International Journal of Vitamins Nutrition and Supplements,* vol. 30 (1989).

Mackenzie, Niall, D.P.M., M.A., et al. "Premenstrual Syndrome and Progesterone Suppositories." (Letter.) *Journal of the American Medical Association,* vol. 265, no. 1 (January 2, 1991).

Magos, A. L. "Effects and Analysis of the Menstrual Cycle." *Journal of Biomedical Engineering,* vol. 10, no. 2 (April 1988).

Mauri, M., et al. "Sleep in the Premenstrual Phase: A Self-Report Study of PMS Patients and Normal Controls." *Acta Psychiatry Scandinavia,* vol. 78, no. 1 (July 1988).

Mello, N. K., et al. "Alcohol Use and Premenstrual Symptoms in Social Drinkers." *Psychopharmacology,* vol. 101, no. 4 (1990).

Messinis, I. E., and D. Lolis. "Treatment of Premenstrual Mastalgia with Tamoxifen." *Acta Obstetricia Gynecologia Scandinavia,* vol. 67, no. 4 (1988).

Metcalf, M. G., et al. "Mood Cyclicity in Women with and Without the Premenstrual Syndrome." *Journal of Psychosomatic Resident,* vol. 33, no. 4 (1989).

Mira, M., et al. "Vitamin and Trace Element Status in Premenstrual Syndrome." *American Journal of Clinical Nutrition,* vol. 47, no. 4 (April 1988).

Mortola, J. F., et al. "Depressive Episodes in Premenstrual Syndrome." *American Journal of Obstetrics and Gynecology,* vol. 161, no. 6, pt. 1 (December 1989).

Nikolai, T. F., et al. "Thyroid Function and Treatment in Premenstrual Syndrome." *Journal of Clinical Endocrinology and Metabolism,* vol. 70, no. 4 (April 1990).

O'Boyle, M., et al. "Premenstrual Syndrome and Locus of

Control." *International Journal of Psychiatry and Medicine,* vol. 18, no. 1 (1988).

Osofsky, Howard J., M.D., Ph.D. "Efficacious Treatments of PMS: A Need for Further Research." *Journal of the American Medical Association,* vol. 264, no. 3 (July 18, 1990).

Pullon, S. R., et al. "Treatment of Premenstrual Symptoms in Wellington Women." *New Zealand Medical Journal,* vol. 102, no. 862 (February 22, 1989).

Quill, T. E., et al. "The Medicalization of Normal Variants." *Journal of General Internal Medicine,* vol. 3, no. 3 (May–June 1988).

Robinson, G. E. "Premenstrual Syndrome: Current Knowledge and Management." *Canadian Medical Association Journal,* vol. 140, no. 6 (March 15, 1989).

————, and P. E. Garfinkel. "Problems in the Treatment of Premenstrual Syndrome." *Canadian Journal of Psychiatry,* vol. 35, no. 3 (April 1990).

Rosen, L. N., et al. "Relationship Between Premenstrual Symptoms and General Well-Being." *Psychosomatics,* vol. 31, no. 1 (Winter 1990).

Rossignol, A. M., and H. Bonnlander. "Caffeine-Containing Beverages, Total Fluid Consumption and Premenstrual Syndrome." *American Journal of Public Health,* vol. 80, no. 9 (September 1990).

Rothbaum, B. O., and J. Jackson. "Religious Influence on Menstrual Attitudes and Symptoms." *Women and Health,* vol. 16, no. 1 (1990).

Rovner, Sandy. "Caffeine Beverages Worsen Premenstrual Symptoms." *The Washington Post,* September 11, 1990.

Rubinow, D. R., et al. "Changes in Plasma Hormones Across the Menstrual Cycle in Patients with Menstrually Related Mood Disorder and in Control Subjects." *Ameri-*

can Journal of Obstetrics and Gynecology, vol. 158, no. 1 (January 1988).

Simpson, L. O. "The Etiopathogenesis of Premenstrual Syndrome as a Consequence of Altered Blood Rheology: A New Hypothesis." *Medical Hypotheses,* vol. 25, no. 4 (April 1988).

————, et al. "Factors Influencing the Cyclical Symptoms Relating to the Menstrual Cycle." *New Zealand Medical Journal,* vol. 101, no. 845 (May 11, 1988).

Silber, M., et al. "Premenstrual Syndrome in a Group of Hysterectomized Women of Reproductive Age with Intact Ovaries." *Advances in Contraception,* vol. 5, no. 3 (September 1989).

Stein, M. B., et al. "Panic Disorder and the Menstrual Cycle." *American Journal of Psychiatry,* vol. 146, no. 10 (October 1989).

Stewart, D. E. "Positive Changes in the Premenstrual Period." *Acta Psychiatria Scandinavia,* vol. 79, no. 4 (April 1989).

Taghavi, E. "Premenstrual Syndrome in Three Generations Responds to Antidepressants." *Australia and New Zealand Journal of Psychiatry,* vol. 24, no. 2 (June 1990).

Toth, A., et al. "Effect of Doxycycline on Premenstrual Syndrome." *Journal of Internal Medicine Residents,* vol. 16, no. 4 (July–August 1988).

Van den Akker, O., and A. Steptoe. "Psychophysiological Responses in Women Reporting Severe Premenstrual Symptoms." *Psychosomatic Medicine,* vol. 51, no. 3 (May–June 1989).

Walker, A., and J. Bancroft. "Relationship Between Premenstrual Symptoms and Oral Contraceptive Use: A Controlled Study." *Psychosomatic Medicine,* vol. 52, no. 1 (January–February 1990).

Warnick, Mark S. "Antidepressant Drug Under Fire." *Rocky Mountain News*, September 5, 1990.

West, C. P. "The Characteristics of 100 Women Presenting to a Gynecological Clinic with Premenstrual Complaints." *Acta Obstetrica Gynecologia Scandinavia*, vol. 68, no. 8 (1989).

———. "Inhibition of Ovulation with Oral Progestins—Effectiveness in Premenstrual Syndrome." *European Journal of Obstetrics Gynecology and Reproductive Biology*, vol. 34, no. 1–2 (January–February 1990).

Wickes, S. L. "Premenstrual Syndrome." *Primary Care*, vol. 15, no. 3 (September 1988).

Wilson, C. A., and W. R. Keye, Jr. "A Survey of Adolescent Dysmenorrhea and Premenstrual Symptom Frequency: A Model Program for Prevention, Detection and Treatment." *Journal of Adolescent Health Care*, vol. 10, no. 4 (July 1989).

Wolf, Michele. "The PMS Diet: Mood-Lifting Weight Loss." *Bazaar* (November 1988).

Wurtman, J. J. "Carbohydrate Craving: Relationship Between Carbohydrate Intake and Disorders of Mood." *Drugs*, vol. 39, supplement 3 (1990).

———, et al. "Effect of Nutrient Intake on Premenstrual Depression." *American Journal of Obstetrics and Gynecology*, vol. 161, no. 5 (November 1989).

Yuk, V. J., et al. "Towards a Definition of PMS: A Factor Analytic Evaluation of Premenstrual Change in Non-Complaining Women." *Journal of Psychosomatic Residency*, vol. 34, no. 4 (1990).

INDEX

ABOUT THE AUTHOR

PAMELA PATRICK NOVOTNY is a journalist whose work has appeared in many newspapers and magazines. Her first book, *The Joy of Twins* (Crown Publishers), was published in 1988. She is also the author of two other books in the Dell Medical Library, *What You Can Do About Infertility* and *What Women Should Know About Chronic Infections and Sexually Transmitted Diseases,* to be published in 1992. She is also at work on a novel. Pamela Patrick Novotny holds a degree in journalism from the University of Colorado, where she also teaches writing. She lives in Colorado with her family.